PIONEERS IN SCIENCE

MEDICINE

PETER LAFFERTY

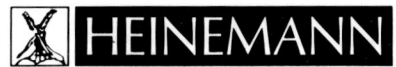

First published in 1992 by
Heinemann Children's Reference,
a division of Heinemann Educational Books Ltd,
Halley Court, Jordan Hill, Oxford OX2 8EJ

96 95 94 93
10 9 8 7 6 5 4 3 2

OXFORD LONDON EDINBURGH
MADRID PARIS ATHENS BOLOGNA
MELBOURNE SYDNEY AUCKLAND SINGAPORE TOKYO
IBADAN NAIROBI GABORONE HARARE
PORTSMOUTH (NH)

Project manager Myra Murby
Editor Mary Melling
Designer Jerry Burman
Picture researchers Catherine Blackie, Suzanne Williams

Printed in Hong Kong

British Library Cataloguing in Publication Data

Lafferty, Peter
    Medicine. – (Pioneers in science)
    1. Medicine, history
    I. Title II. Series
    610.9

ISBN 0-431-00794-2

Photographic acknowledgements

t=top b=bottom r=right l=left c=centre

The Bridgeman Art Library/Weston Park, Shropshire 14; Bridgeman Art library 17b, 20, 24; Bridgeman Art Library/ City of York Art Gallery, anon 17th c. Dutch school, *The Doctor's Shop* 34; C. M. Dixon 6b; E. T. Archive/St Mary's Hospital Medical School 37l; Sally & Richard Greenhill 27b, 41; Michael Holford 7, 21b, 28b; The Hulton Picture Company 8t, 12l, 16, 26; The Hutchison Library/Juliet Rasmussen 40b; London School of Hygiene and Tropical medicine 30l; The Mansell Collection 9, 25b; Mary Evans Picture Library 6t, 10l & r, 12r, 15l, 17t, 18, 19t, 19b, 21t, 22, 23t, 32, 35l, 39t; Peter Newark's Pictures 27t; The Florence Nightingale Museum Trust 25t; Oxford Scientific Films/Tim Shepherd 30r; Popperfoto 36; Rex Features 42tr; Medical Illustration Unit, Royal college of Surgeons 29; Science Photo Library 13, 15r, 23b, 28t, 35r; Science Photo Library/Jerry Mason 33t & b; Science Photo Library/ Lawrence Malvehill 37r; Science Photo Library/Hank Morgan 42bl, 43; Frank Spooner Pictures 5; Topham Picture source/Associated Press 40t; Miriam Mc Curdy 39b; World Health Organization 31; Reproduced by kind permission of the Dean and Chapter of York: Photographer – Peter Gibson 4.

Cover: Bridgeman Art Library l, c; Popperfoto r; The Florence Nightingale Museum Trust b.
Cover pictures show: Florence Nightingale l; Louis Pasteur c; Alexander Fleming r; Painting of Florencs Nightingale in the military hospital at Scutari b.

Note to the reader
In this book there are some words in the text that are printed in bold type. This shows that the word is listed in the glossary on page 46. The glossary gives a brief explanation of words that may be new to you.

Contents

The beginnings of medicine

People today do not die from toothache or a slight cold. Ancient civilizations, however, knew very little about how to cure illness and **disease**. They often relied on magic to treat the sick. Five thousand years ago, one of the first great civilizations flourished in Egypt. Egyptian priests thought that sickness was sent by the gods to punish men and women for their sins. These priests prayed to the gods to help the sick and to fight off evil spirits.

To cure blindness, they mashed up the eye of a pig and poured it into the blind person's ear! These treatments could not have had much success.

Two early doctors

Discoveries about the way the body works and about how to cure disease have gradually been made over the past 2000 years by many doctors and scientists. The first great doctor was a

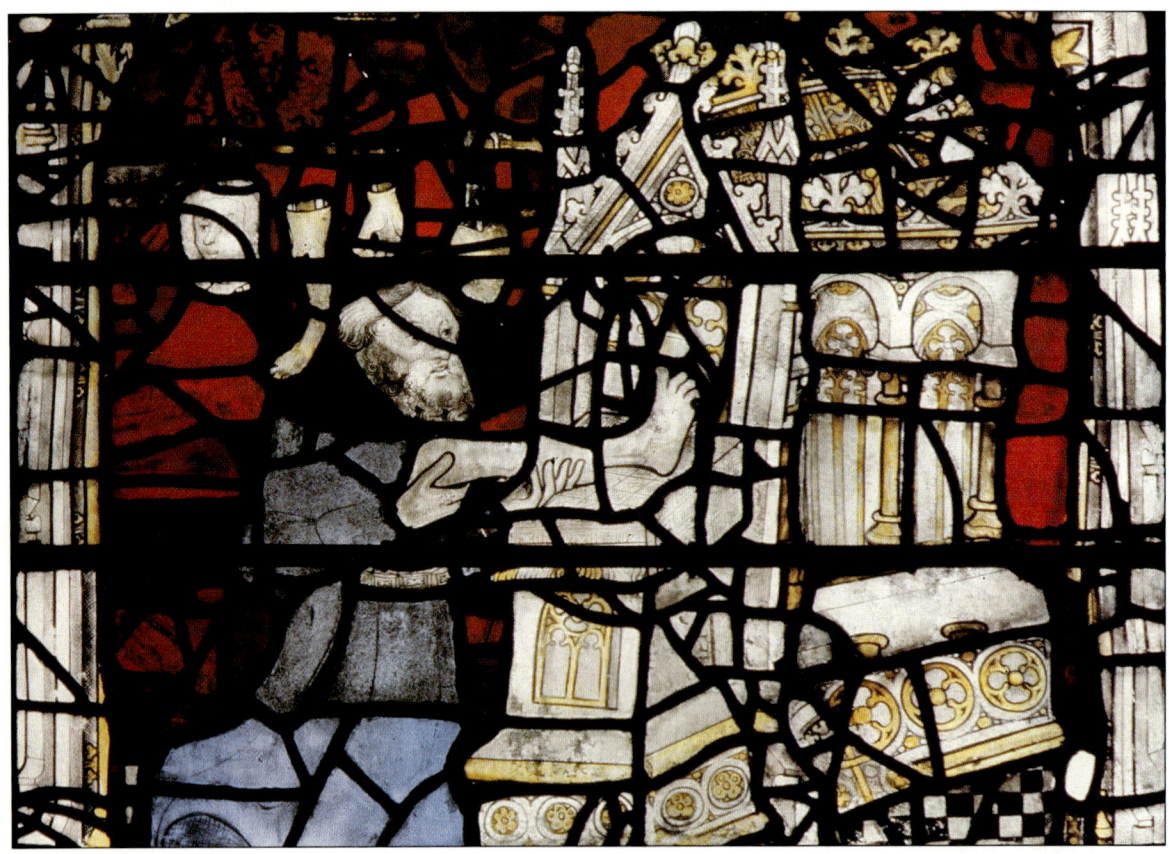

Praying for a cure. This window from York Minster shows a man offering a wax model of his leg to the shrine of St. William in hope of a cure. Even today, pilgrims visit holy places, such as Lourdes in France, seeking cures. For most people, modern medicine offers a better chance.

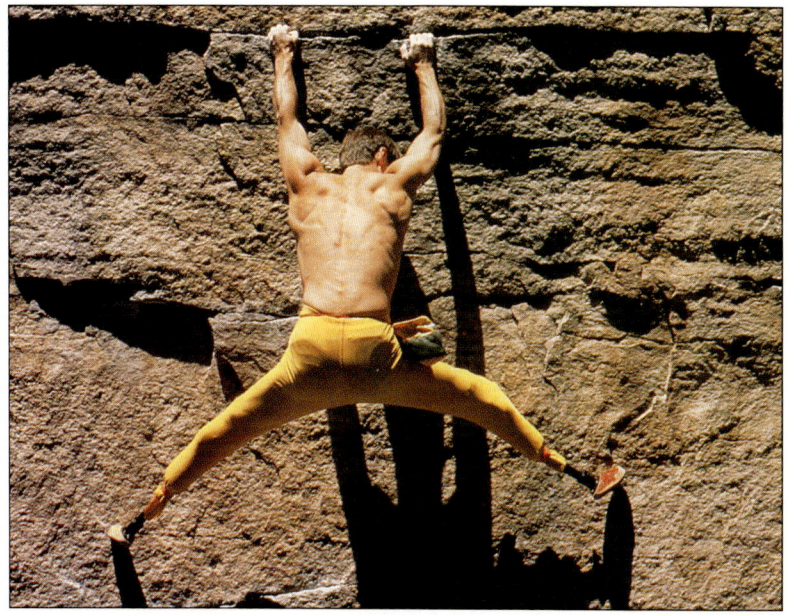

Mountain climbing without legs. This young man lost both legs in an accident. Modern artificial legs contain electronics so that they 'feel' like a natural leg. Now disabled people can walk, run and even climb if they want to.

Greek called Hippocrates. He insisted on looking carefully at a sick person, to see exactly what was wrong before trying to cure them. He realized that sickness was not sent by the gods and that it had a natural cause.

Another great doctor was called Galen. He lived in Rome about 1800 years ago. He discovered that many diseases are caused by damage in the body. However, he had a very common fault. He was certain that everything he said was true. He was so confident, that even other people came to believe that he could not be mistaken. Of course, he did make mistakes but it was over 1000 years before his mistakes were discovered.

The ideas of Hippocrates and Galen spread to the Arab world but were almost forgotten in Europe. For this reason, for over 600 years, Arab doctors were the best in the world. However, in the 14th and 15th centuries, doctors in Europe began to study books written by Hippocrates and Galen again.

From magic to science

As time went on, medicine became a **science**. Doctors began doing experiments to test their ideas and they collected as much information about diseases as they could. In this way, the mistakes of Galen and Hippocrates were discovered and corrected. Scientists have found how many diseases are caused by small organisms, called **bacteria** or **germs**. They have developed many effective medicines, or **drugs**, to kill bacteria, and ways of removing diseased parts of the body without pain. Now it is even possible to replace some parts of the body. This book tells the stories of some of those men and women who have made modern medicine possible.

5

The father of modern medicine

Over 2500 years ago, the ancient Greeks believed that illness was caused by the gods. Their doctors were priests who prayed to the gods for healing. The most important god of healing was called Asclepius and temples called Asclepaeia were built to worship him. These temples were also used as hospitals where the priests treated sick people. The sick person, or **patient**, was given poppy seeds to make them sleep. When the person was asleep, the priests performed a ceremony to heal them. Some people seem to have been cured in this way, because they believed in the priest's powers.

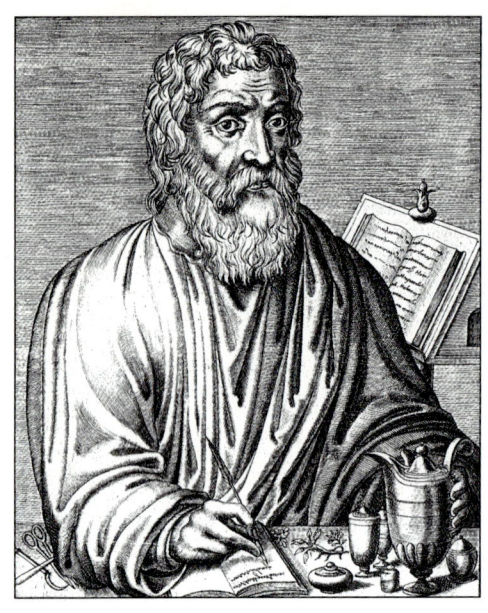

▲ **Hippocrates, the father of modern medicine**. Hippocrates lived about 2400 years ago, but his ideas are still important. Until recently all new doctors swore an oath to help their patients and to behave properly. The oath was called the 'Hippocratic Oath' because Hippocrates first used it.

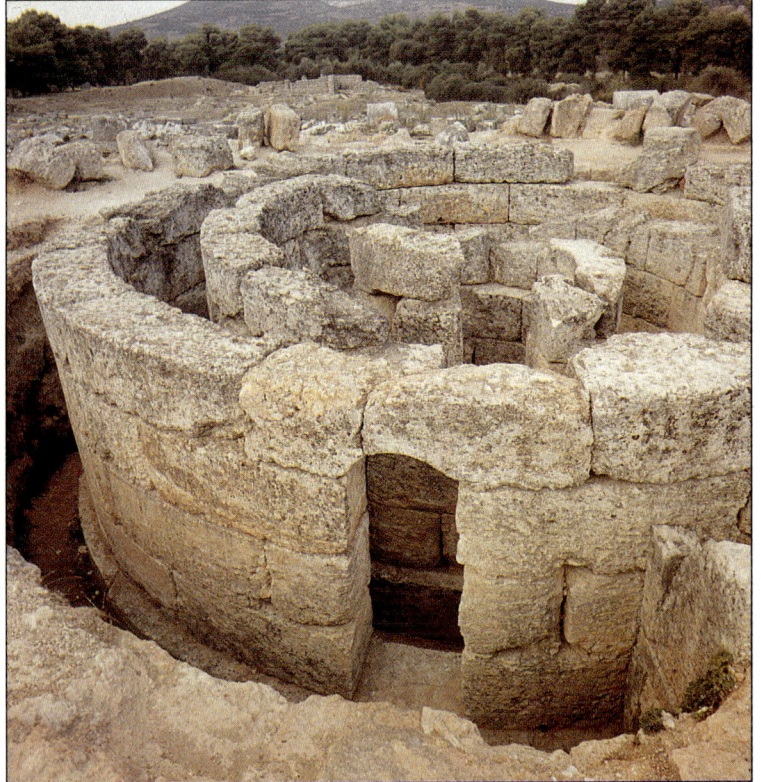

◄ **A Greek temple of healing dedicated to Asclepius**. The Tholos temple was built about 320 AD at Epidauros. It is said that people came to sleep and have healing dreams in the maze of passages. Others think that the passages were for sacred snakes which were put on a sleeping person to lick the wounds.

Hippocrates

About 2400 years ago, a Greek doctor called Hippocrates began to question the old ways of treating sick people. Hippocrates was born on the island of Cos, near the coast of Turkey. He travelled widely to places such as Egypt to study and teach medicine. Eventually he returned to Cos to start a school for doctors.

Hippocrates was the first doctor to realize that diseases are not caused by the gods. He said that they had a natural cause and that if a doctor understood a disease, it could be treated. This is the way we treat illness today, and so Hippocrates is called the 'father of modern medicine'.

Four stages and four liquids

Hippocrates taught that, to cure a sick person, a doctor should do four things. First of all, the doctor must examine the patient carefully, to see what is wrong. Next, the doctor must decide what is likely to happen as the illness progresses. The doctor should then watch and write down what happens. Finally, if necessary, the doctor should give some treatment to cure the illness. Hippocrates made careful notes about each disease he saw and kept records of the health of each patient. He found that with rest and good food, the body could often cure itself. More than a hundred years after he died, his ideas were written down in a collection of books called the 'Hippocratic Collection'. These books

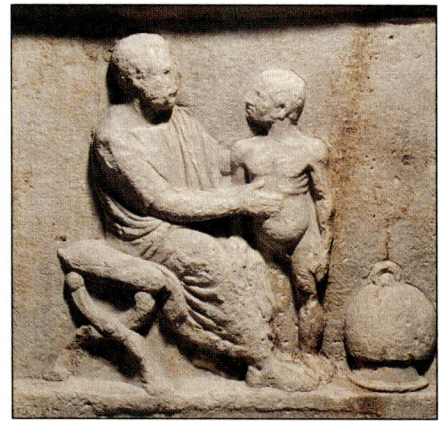

A Greek doctor examines a patient. This carving from a Greek tomb shows a doctor and a patient. Greek doctors realized that it was important to examine a patient carefully before prescribing treatment. This is part of the 'modern' approach to medicine first used by Hippocrates.

helped to spread his ideas to other countries.

Some of Hippocrates' ideas were wrong. He believed that the body contained four 'humours' or liquids, called blood, phlegm, yellow bile and black bile. A person was only healthy if the right amounts of each humour were present in the body. The patient's treatment depended upon which humour was present in the wrong amount. If the patient was spitting blood, it meant that there was too much blood in the body. So a small cut was made to let the extra blood out.

Although Hippocrates spent a lot of time observing illness, he did not believe in cutting up, or **dissecting**, dead human bodies. As a result, he did not know much about the inside of the body. Nevertheless, his method of working and his ideas started a more scientific way of treating illness.

The gladiators' doctor

Claudius Galen was another important doctor of ancient times. He was born in AD130, in the town of Pergamon in the country now called Turkey. In Galen's time, this was a part of Greece ruled by the Romans. To please his father, he studied to be a doctor. When he was 20 years old, he set out to visit the main medical schools in Greece, Egypt and other parts of the Roman Empire. For nine years he travelled widely, learning all he could.

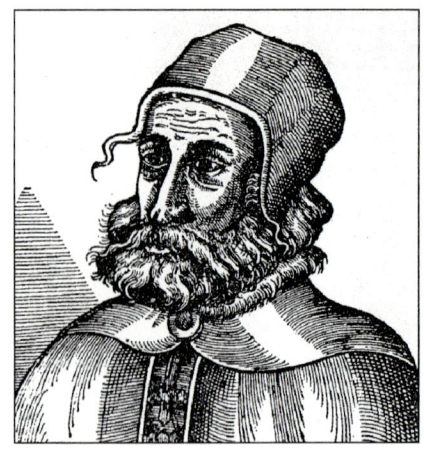

▲ Galen (130–200), the most famous doctor in the Roman world. Like Hippocrates, he believed in carefully studying what was wrong before treating a sick person.

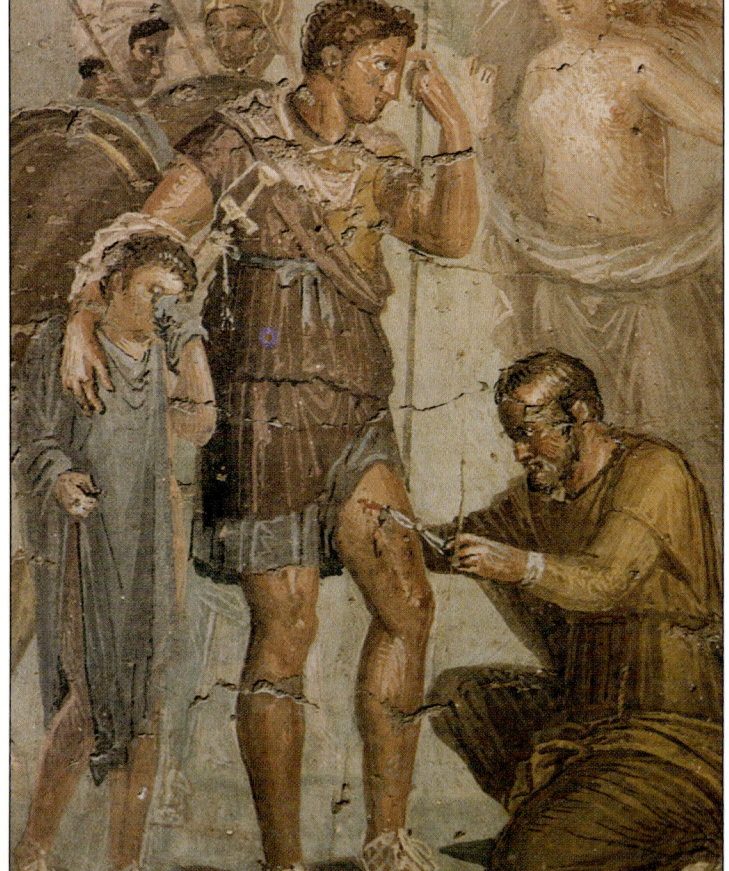

◀ **Treating a wounded gladiator.** This wall painting from the Roman city of Pompei shows a gladiator having a cut treated by a Roman doctor, perhaps Galen. The gladiator's companion seems more upset than the gladiator.

When he returned to Pergamon he became the doctor at a school for gladiators, men who fought each other to entertain the crowds at festivals. This job helped him study the human body because the gladiators were often cut and wounded in their fights.

Learning from animals

His work with the gladiators taught him that deep cuts and wounds often left the injured person unable to move. From this he guessed that many diseases were caused by injuries to the body. However, at this time it was forbidden to cut up, or dissect, human bodies because the Romans believed that dead people needed their bodies for life after death. This made it difficult for Galen to learn how cuts and injuries affected the human body, so he tried to find out as much as possible by dissecting animals. He performed many experiments on animals, such as pigs, dogs and apes, and even a hippopotamus and an elephant.

Ideas about the heart

In the year 161 Galen went to Rome. There he became famous after he cured the ruler of Rome of a stomach ache. He wrote more than 300 books, and other doctors used his ideas. Some of them are still used today. For example, he was the first doctor to take the pulse of his patients, like modern doctors do.

Unfortunately, some of his ideas were wrong, because the bodies of the animals he studied are different from human bodies. For example, he was wrong about the way the heart works. Galen thought that there were two separate flows of blood in the body. He thought that one flow of blood travelled from the heart to some parts of the body and then back to the heart, and the other flow of blood went from the heart to the rest of the body. However, for many hundreds of years Galen's ideas were considered to be very important. More than 1300 years later, in 1539, a doctor in London was made to apologize when he suggested that Galen might be wrong.

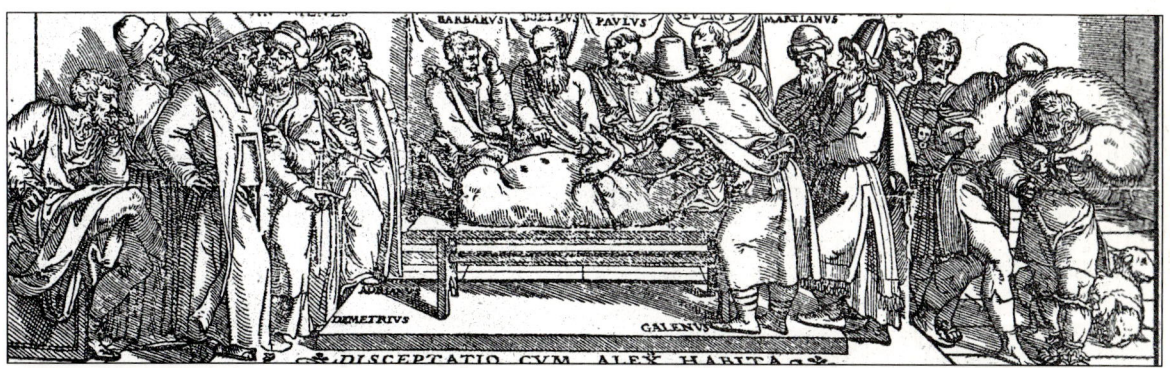

Galen dissecting a pig. In Roman times, it was against the law to cut up human bodies to study them. So Galen cut up animals such as pigs. He made many discoveries but, because a human body is different from the body of an animal, he made mistakes too.

Towards modern surgery

Surgery is the performing of an operation to cure a disease or to heal a wound. Until the 1500s surgery was only done by a few doctors, or by barbers who spent most of their time cutting hair. The main operations were tooth-pulling, and cutting off diseased legs or arms. These operations were very painful and dangerous. There were no pain-killing drugs and many patients died because of the great pain of the operation. The surgeons often used dirty instruments, which caused wounds to become swollen and rotten. The first person to introduce better, safer methods was Ambroise Paré.

Heat treatment for wounds

Ambroise Paré had little education. He started his medical career as a barber's assistant where he learned enough to get a job as a wound dresser at the Hôtel-Dieu, a famous hospital in Paris. In

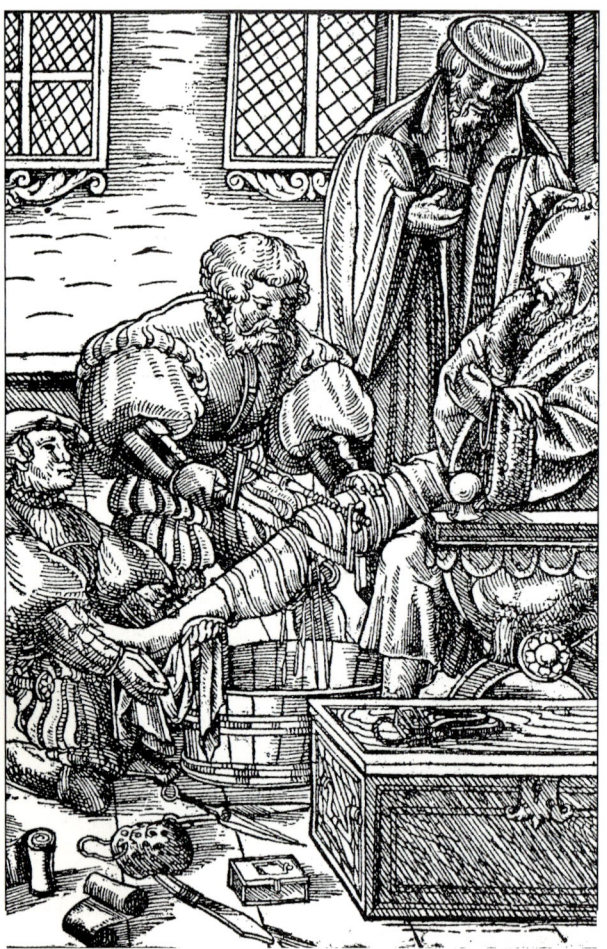

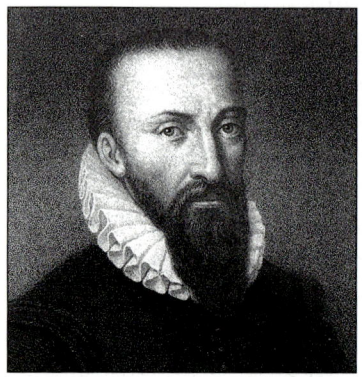

▲ **Ambroise Paré (1510–90)**, a great French surgeon, was the first doctor in Europe to tie the ends of cut blood vessels, instead of treating them with a red hot iron, to stop bleeding.

◀ **Cutting off a diseased leg, around 1500.** There were no strong pain-killing drugs, so patients were knocked unconcious before an operation. A priest stands by, as many people died during these operations. Paré introduced many improved methods which made surgery less frightening and dangerous.

1537 he became a surgeon in the French army and for the next 20 years he treated soldiers who were wounded while fighting in wars.

In those days, wounds were treated by pouring boiling oil on them, or by pressing a very hot iron onto the wound. This was done to stop the wound going bad and festering. It was very painful and often the wound would swell up. One day, the oil Paré was using became too thick to boil and he was forced to try another method. He made up a mixture of egg yolks and cool thick oil and put the mixture on a gunshot wound. That night, he could not sleep because he was worried that the soldier would die. However, to his surprise, the soldier did not die and the wound healed more quickly than wounds treated with boiling oil. From then on, he gave up using boiling oil and heated irons.

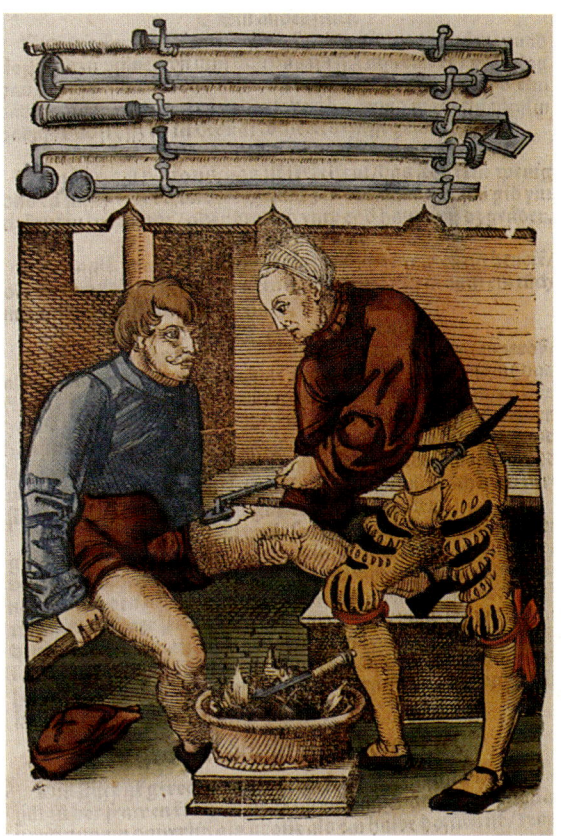

Treating a gunshot wound, medieval style. In the Middle Ages, around 1500, wounds were treated with a very hot iron or boiling oil. This stopped the bleeding but was very painful.

More improved methods

Paré discovered other new ways to treat wounds. In order to stop the loss of blood during operations, he began to tie blood vessels with string. This was better than the usual method of using a heated iron. He also made artificial legs for people who had lost a leg through disease or injury.

He made new tools for surgeons to use and wrote books to show surgeons how to improve their work. For a while, his discoveries were ignored by some doctors. They did not believe what he said because he did not write his books in Latin. At that time all educated people wrote in Latin rather than their own language. Eventually, however, his methods were used all over France. He became surgeon to the king, and served the royal family for many years. Paré's improvements had made surgery a less frightening and more successful method of treatment.

The body snatcher

Andreas Vesalius was born in 1514 in Brussels. As a young boy, he was fascinated by the way animals' bodies were made. He would cut open dead mice, birds and other small animals so that he could see their muscles, bones and organs. Later, he became a medical student and studied the human body. He used to steal the bodies of criminals after they had been executed. He took the bodies apart, then he soaked the bones in vinegar to hide the smell and smuggled them into his room to study them. He was a brilliant student and was soon made a professor at the University of Padua, which was an important medical school in Italy.

Challenging old ideas

Vesalius was a popular teacher and hundreds of students would come to his classes. He used to show what he was talking about by cutting up a body

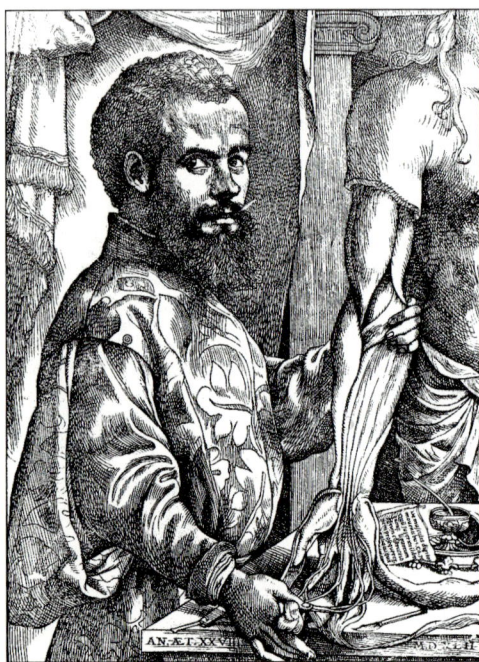

Andreas Vesalius (1514–64), who started the scientific study of the human body. This Belgian doctor settled in the Italian town of Padua where he taught anatomy, the study of the human body. Hundreds of pupils attended his lectures. He always dissected a body as he talked, to show what he meant. Other teachers just read aloud from a book and left the dissection to an assistant.

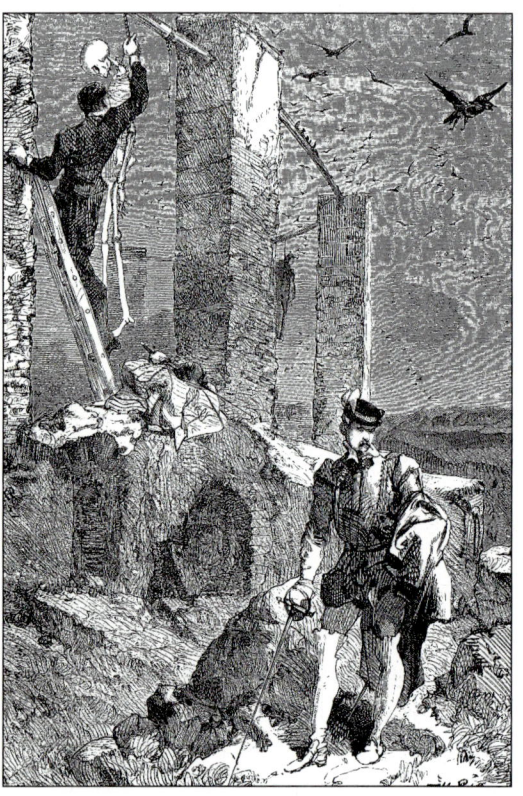

The body snatcher. Andreas Vesalius realized how important it is to dissect the human body to find out how it is made. But it was not easy to find bodies to study. Here Vesalius steals the body of an executed criminal from the gallows.

during his lectures. He also used large charts and diagrams to help his pupils understand. He told his students to study the human body for themselves, and not to believe what they read in old medical books.

At that time, all medical schools taught the ideas of Galen, the doctor of ancient Rome. However, Galen had only studied animals, not people. Vesalius soon found that Galen was sometimes wrong. For example, Galen had said that human beings had two bones in the jaw. Vesalius found that the human jaw is formed of a single bone. He also found that men and women have the same number of ribs. This was a surprise because the Church taught that God had taken a rib from Adam, the first man, to make the first woman, Eve. So men were supposed to have less ribs than women.

Showing what is inside a body

In 1543 Vesalius wrote a book showing what he had discovered about the body. The book was called *The Structure of the Human Body* and it was the first book to describe the inside of the human body accurately. It contained many large and detailed diagrams of the muscles, nerves and blood vessels of the body. His book started a whole new science, called **anatomy**. This is the science that studies how the human body is constructed.

Unfortunately, Vesalius's success and popularity made other doctors jealous. They attacked him for saying that Galen

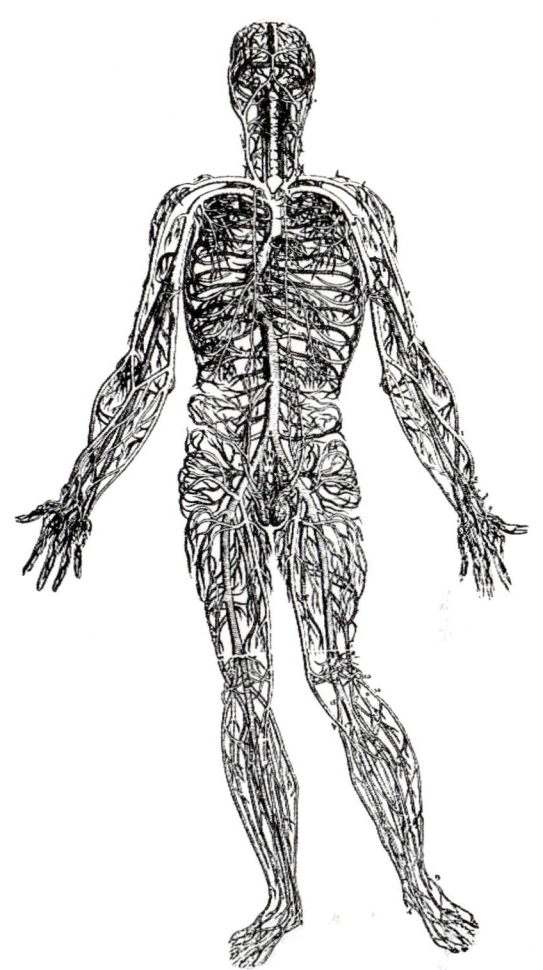

Inside the body. A drawing of the human blood vessels made by Vesalius. In 1543, Vesalius published a book, called *The Structure of the Human Body*, which contained the first pictures of how the body is constructed.

was wrong. Partly because of this, Vesalius left Padua and became the doctor to the emperor Charles V of Spain. At the age of 50 he was sent on a trip to the Holy Land, as a punishment for stealing bodies. On the way home, his ship was wrecked and he drowned, but his pioneering work in finding out how the human body is made helped many other doctors improve medical science.

How blood flows

One of Galen's ideas was that there are two types of blood in the body. Bright red blood was carried by blood vessels, called **arteries**. Dark red blood was carried by **veins**. Galen thought that the two types of blood were completely separate. He thought that blood flowed back and forth in the arteries and veins. The man who proved him wrong was William Harvey. He was able to show that the heart pumps blood around the body in a continuous loop, through the arteries, into the veins, then back to the heart.

A one-way system

William Harvey was born in 1578, in Folkestone, England. In 1598 he went to study medicine at the University of Padua, in Italy. There, his teacher was Hieronymous Fabricius. Fabricius had discovered that veins contained one-way valves, which meant that blood could only flow in one direction in the veins, towards the heart. This discovery puzzled Harvey. He wondered what happened to the blood after it had flowed along the veins.

After returning to England, Harvey settled in London. He obtained work at St Bartholomew's hospital, the only hospital in the city of London. Later, he joined the College of Physicians, an important society of doctors. He continued to think about the way blood flowed in the body and he did experiments to check how the valves in

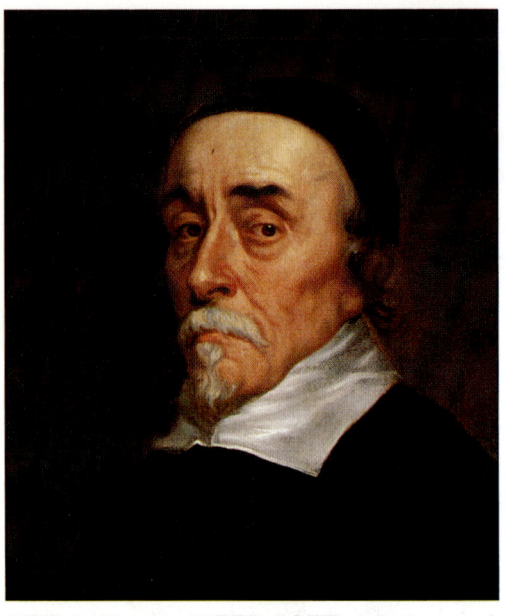

William Harvey (1578–1657), who around 1616 discovered how the blood circulates in our bodies. It took many years for doctors to accept Harvey's ideas.

blood vessels worked. He dissected a human heart and found that it was a one-way pump. He also found that the arteries always carried blood away from the heart, never towards it.

A circular flow

Harvey worked out how much blood his own heart pumped in an hour. To his surprise, he found that the amount of blood pumped was equal to three times the weight of his whole body. The only way this could happen was if the same blood was being pumped round and round the body. He decided that there must be very fine blood vessels, which were too fine to see, connecting the veins and arteries. Blood flows from the heart along the arteries. Then it passes through very fine blood vessels to the veins and returns to the heart. This circular flow is called the **circulation** of the blood.

Harvey wrote down his ideas in a book in 1628. There was a storm of protests and criticism. Many doctors could not believe that Galen was wrong. However, by the time Harvey died in 1657, most doctors thought he was right. He had made a major discovery about the human body.

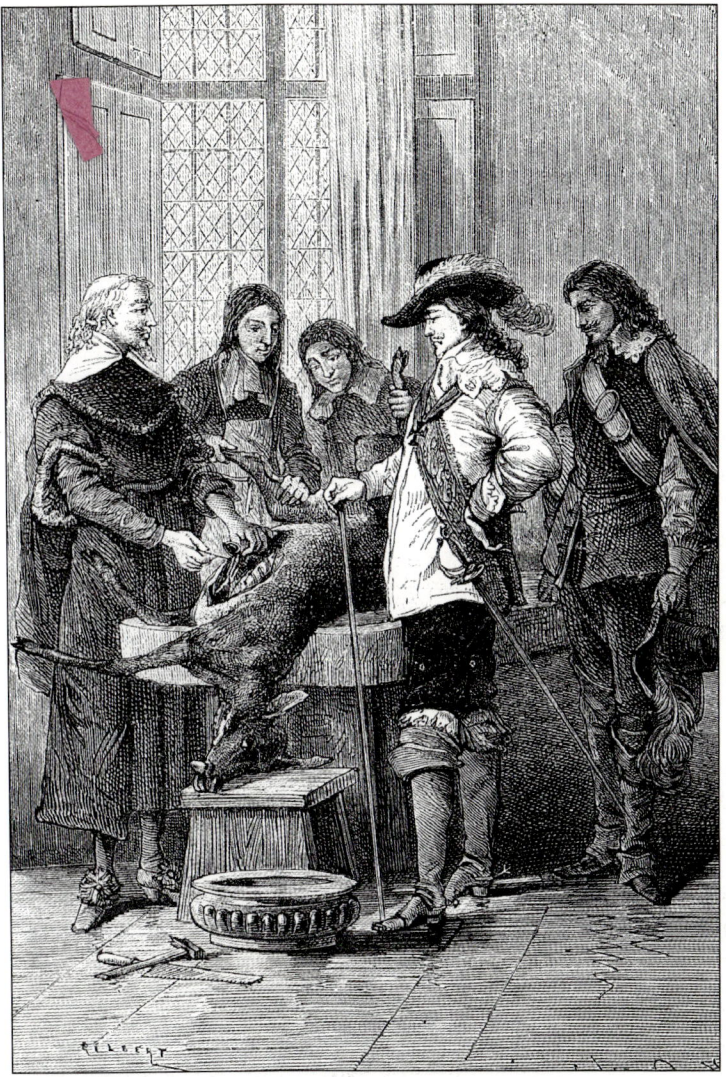

The royal doctor. William Harvey became doctor to King James I and later to Charles I. Here Harvey shows King Charles I how the blood circulates in the body of a deer. The future King Charles II looks on.

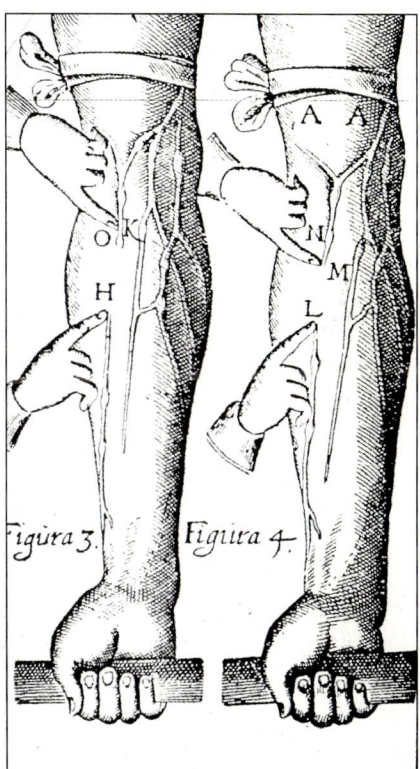

▲ **One-way system.** This picture, from Harvey's book *On the Motions of the Heart and Blood*, shows an experiment to prove that blood only flows one way in the veins. The small bulges in the veins are valves. When a finger is pressed onto a vein, and moved towards the wrist, blood empties out of a section of the vein. The valve stops the blood flowing from the upper arm and filling the vein.

Preventing disease

Nobody gets smallpox now, but 200 years ago it was one of the most feared diseases. Smallpox caused spots and blisters to break out all over the body and was passed easily from one person to another. Smallpox killed 60 million people in Europe in the years between 1700 and 1800. In bad years, one person out of three died of the disease. Those that survived the disease were left with horrible scars, and were often blinded. Today, smallpox has been wiped out thanks to a discovery by an English doctor called Edward Jenner.

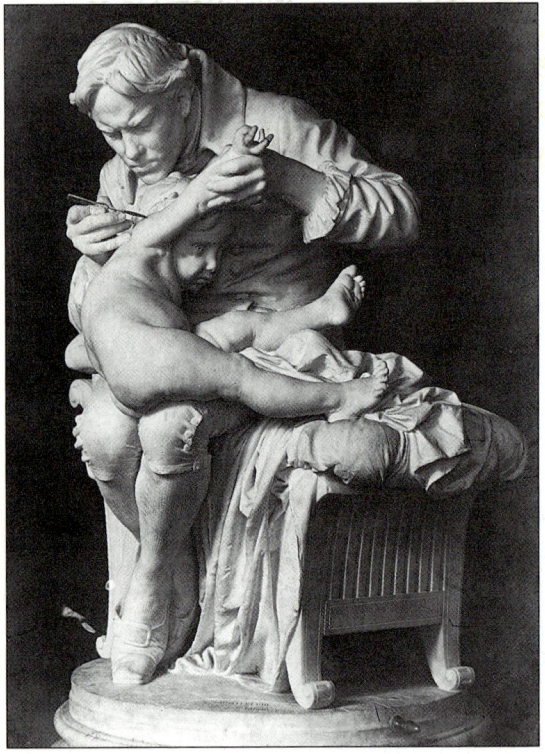

The first vaccination. The sculpture shows Edward Jenner vaccinating eight-year-old James Phipps against smallpox. This risky experiment was the start of a great medical success story.

The country doctor

Edward Jenner was born in Berkeley, in Gloucestershire, England, in 1749. He studied medicine in London with John Hunter, a famous surgeon. Then he worked as a doctor in a village near Bristol, in the west of England. A local dairymaid told him that a person who caught cowpox would not catch smallpox. That person was immune to, or protected against, smallpox. Cowpox is a skin disease, similar to smallpox, that is caught from cows but it is not a serious disease. Dairymaids were glad to get cowpox because it seemed to stop them getting smallpox. Jenner wondered if this story was true so he decided to do an experiment to check it.

A dangerous experiment

In May 1796 Jenner took some liquid from the sores on the hand of a dairymaid, Sarah Nelmes, who had cowpox. He then made two small cuts in the arm of an eight-year-old boy called James Phipps. Next, Jenner put the liquid from the sores into the cuts. Naturally, young James caught cowpox, but this is a mild disease and he soon recovered. A few weeks later, Jenner did the same thing, but with liquid taken from a smallpox sore. This was a very risky action because James could have died if he had caught smallpox. Jenner would then have been guilty of murder and would probably have been hanged.

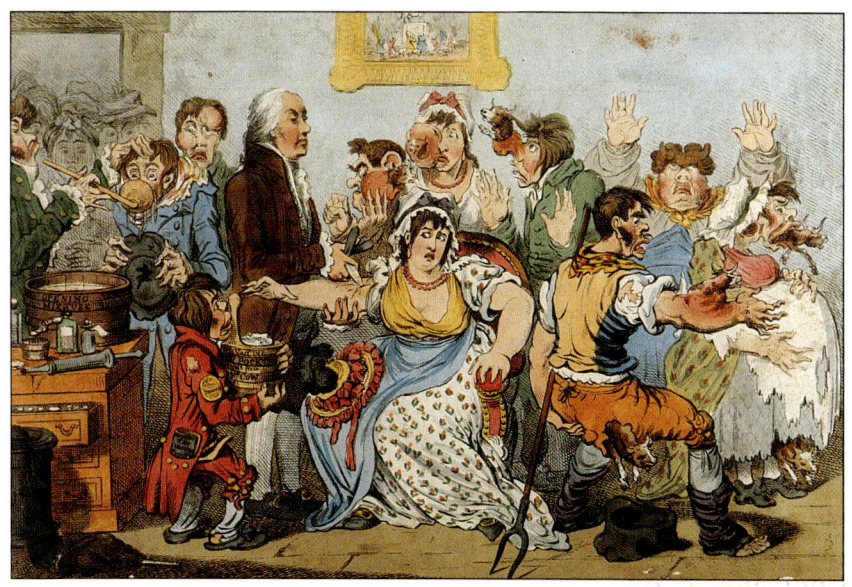

Luckily, James remained healthy.

Later, Jenner repeated the experiment on other people. As before, the experiments were successful. He found that the treatment protected people against smallpox. In 1798, he announced his results. Jenner's treatment was called **vaccination**. The word vaccination comes from *vacca*, the Latin word for cow. At first, people did not like the idea of being injected with fluid from a cow.

Setting a royal example

Nevertheless, the treatment became popular when members of the British royal family were vaccinated. Many people then came to Jenner to be vaccinated and the number of deaths from smallpox dropped rapidly. Jenner was honoured by parliament and given money to carry on his experiments. He died in in 1823, in Berkeley, the village where he was born.

Less than 200 years after Jenner's death, the treatment of smallpox had become so successful that no new cases of it were seen anywhere in the world. Jenner's discovery also led to different sorts of vaccination. If a doctor or nurse injects a small amount of disease germs into us, our bodies can produce chemicals known as **antibodies**, which help fight the germ and so prevent us from becoming ill. Today we can be vaccinated to protect ourselves from many diseases that would have been fatal years ago.

17

Painless surgery

Today, millions of people have operations every year. Most of them feel no pain at all and recover quickly. In the early days of surgery, however, an operation was a dangerous and painful experience. There were no pain-killing drugs and many patients died because of the terrible pain of the operation. People having an operation often had to be held still, and had to bite a leather strap to stop their screams. Some people refused to have operations, preferring to die of their illness rather than endure the pain of the operation.

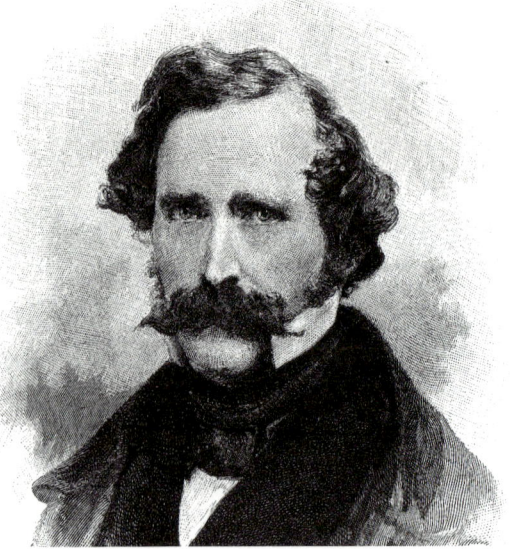

William Morton (1819–68), pioneer of anaesthetics. On October 16, 1846, Morton successfully removed a growth from a young man's jaw using ether as an anaesthetic. When he tried to claim ether as his own invention, to make money from the new discovery, public opinion turned against him. He died, rejected and in poverty, in 1868.

Laughing away the pain

Some pain-killing drugs, or **anaesthetics**, had been known since ancient times but they were not very effective. In 1799 an English chemist called Humphry Davy discovered a gas, which was nicknamed laughing gas. This gas eased pain when it was breathed in. In 1844 an American dentist called Horace Wells used laughing gas to pull out teeth painlessly. The trouble with laughing gas was that it made patients laugh uncontrollably and it did not always put them to sleep during the operation.

The first good anaesthetic was a chemical called **ether**, which put the patient to sleep and killed pain during an operation. This was used by an American doctor, Crawford Long, to painlessly remove a lump from a patient

in 1842. The same year, another American, called William Clark, used ether to pull out a tooth. However, ether did not become widely used until 1846. In that year, an American dentist called William Morton used ether to perform operations in front of an audience of doctors and dentists. News of the discovery spread quickly. Soon doctors all over the world were using ether in their operations.

Unscientific testing

James Simpson was a professor at the University of Edinburgh when he heard of the discovery of ether. He started to use it in his operations but he was not

James Simpson's dangerous experiments. Scottish professor, James Simpson, looking for a better anaesthetic, tested new chemicals on himself. When he first tried chloroform, he quickly became unconscious. On waking, he realized that chloroform was a much better anaesthetic than ether.

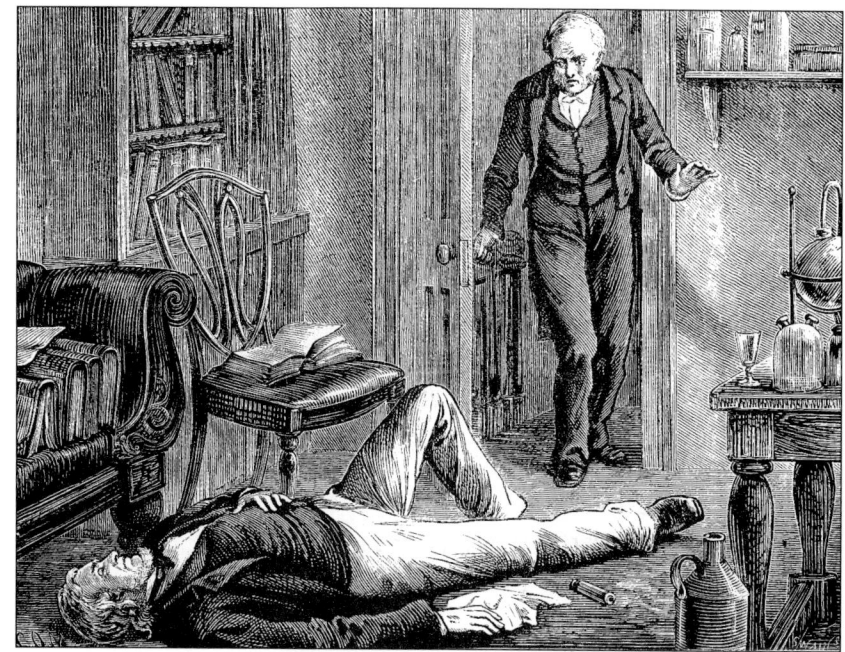

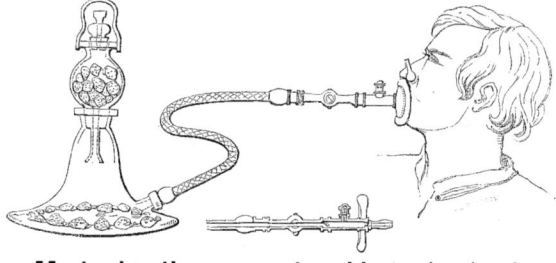

Morton's ether apparatus. Morton's simple device consisted of a glass bottle containing sponges. Ether was poured through the top of the bottle onto the sponges. The patient breathed the ether vapour through an outlet at the side.

completely satisfied with it. Ether had an unpleasant smell and caused the patients to vomit. So he looked for a better pain-killer. Simpson had a dangerous and unscientific way of testing new drugs. He simply sniffed different chemicals to see what effect they had!

One night in 1847 he and two friends sniffed a chemical called **chloroform**. Simpson later wrote, 'The night I took chloroform, Doctor Duncan, Doctor Keith and I all took it at the same time, and we were under the table in a minute or two. When I woke up, I thought "This is better and stronger than ether." Doctor Duncan was asleep under a chair and Doctor Keith was lying on the table, kicking his legs in the air.

Soon Simpson was using chloroform in his operations. Some people objected to the use of chloroform. They said that pain was God's will. However, in 1853, Queen Victoria used chloroform when she had a baby. She said that it was 'soothing, quieting, and delightful beyond all measure.' This convinced the doubters and chloroform became widely used. The successful development of painkillers such as chloroform meant that more and more operations could be carried out safely and successfully and fewer patients died.

Germs and disease

Almost everyone drinks pasteurized milk, but why is milk called 'pasteurized'? The word comes from the name of the scientist who invented the process. He was called Louis Pasteur. Pasteur discovered how germs cause diseases. He was born in Dôle, in France in 1822. He studied science and he became a professor of chemistry when he was only 29 years old. One of his first discoveries was that a very small rod-shaped plant, so small that it could only been seen through a microscope, caused milk to go sour. He also discovered that decay was caused by small microscopic animals, called bacteria or germs, that were carried about by the air.

How to kill germs

Pasteur soon discovered that some germs can cause disease. At that time the silk industry was very important in France and the worms used to produce the silk threads were suffering from a mysterious disease. This was very serious so Pasteur was asked to find out the cause of the disease.

Pasteur found that germs were making the silkworms die and he found a way to prevent the disease. In 1860 he also helped the French wine industry by finding a way to kill off the germs in wine that made it go bad. Pasteur's method was to heat the wine until the germs were killed. This is the process called **pasteurization** that is used today to kill germs in milk.

Preventing killer diseases

Pasteur also studied diseases that affected animals. He soon found that germs were the cause of these diseases, too. He began to look for **vaccines**, which are substances that can be used to prevent diseases. He thought that if he could weaken the germs that were causing a disease, he might be able to make a vaccine out of the weakened germs. After many experiments, he

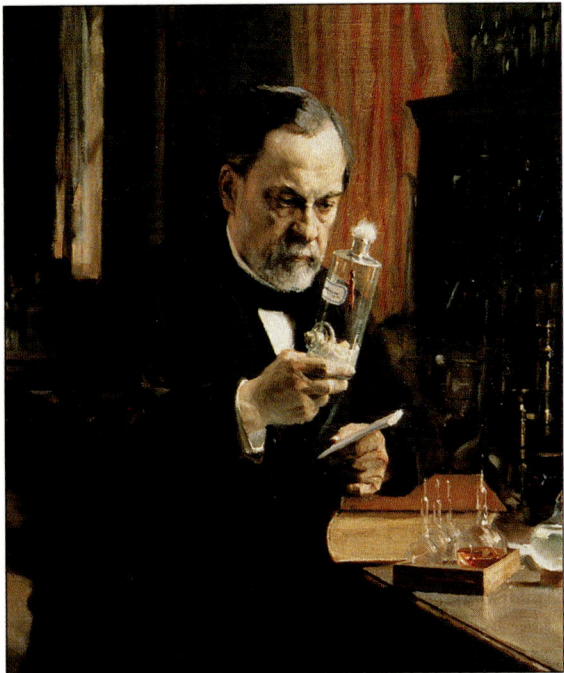

Louis Pasteur (1822–95). Pasteur's discovery that germs cause disease was one of the most important of all time. Here in his laboratory in Paris, the tools of his trade are shown on the bench: sealed flasks containing disease-carrying germs, bottles of vaccine, a microscope.

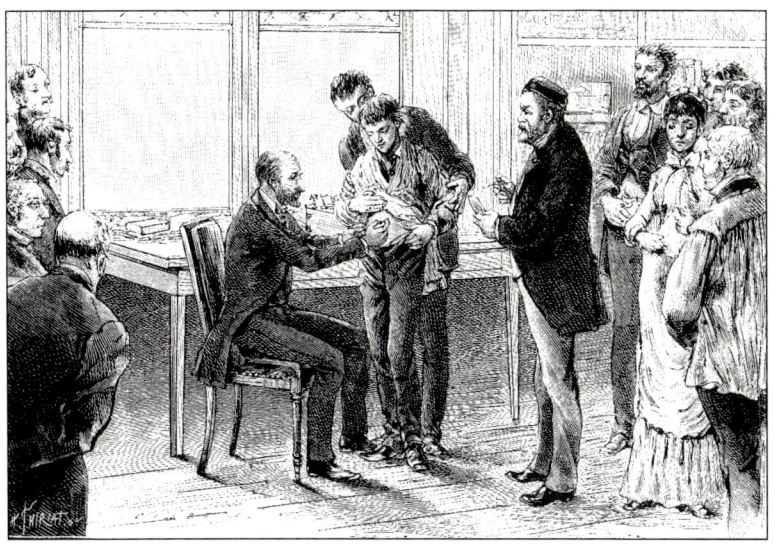

◄ **Pasteur treats Joseph Meister for rabies**. In 1885, a shepherd boy called Joseph Meister became the first person to be treated for rabies by Pasteur, on the right wearing a cap. Rabies can only be cured if the victim is given a vaccine before showing signs of the disease.

▼ **Pasteurizing milk**. Milk is pasteurized by heating it in this machine, for a short time, which kills any germs. Pasteur originally invented the process to improve wines and beers but today it is used for many products, including eggs and cheese.

discovered that some germs that had been kept for a time became weak. These old germs could then be used as a vaccine. Soon Pasteur had developed vaccines that protected chickens and cattle against diseases, such as **anthrax**.

Another disease that Pasteur studied was **rabies**. This is a frightening disease that causes madness and death in dogs and other animals. It also kills people who are bitten by an infected animal. There used to be no way to cure someone who had been infected with the disease. In 1885 Pasteur developed a vaccine, but he was afraid to try it out on a healthy person because it might have given that person the disease.

A household name

One day, however, a nine-year-old boy, called Joseph Meister, was brought to him. Joseph had been bitten by a dog with rabies and he would die if nothing was done, so Pasteur treated him with

the rabies vaccine. Joseph did not die, and Pasteur knew the vaccine was a success.

Pasteur was now famous. In 1888 the French government built a laboratory for him in Paris, called the Pasteur Institute, so that he could continue his work. He worked at the Institute until he died in 1895. The Pasteur Institute has carried on Pasteur's work and it is now an international centre for research into the causes and prevention of disease.

Fighting common diseases

Pasteur's discovery that germs cause some diseases encouraged many other scientists to study bacteria. A hundred years ago, two very serious diseases were **tuberculosis** and **cholera**. Tuberculosis was a common cause of death all over the world and cholera killed thousands of people whenever an outbreak occurred. In 1849 an outbreak of cholera killed 72 000 people in the slums of London. Five years later, another outbreak killed 20 000 people.

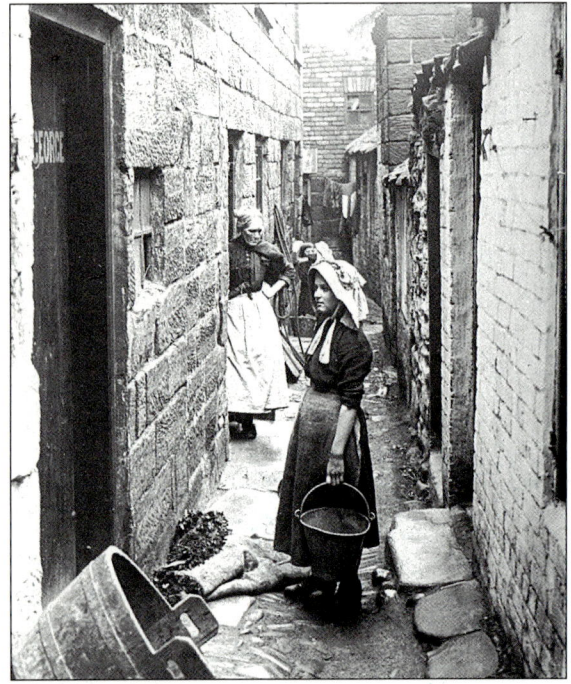

Cholera in the slums. Cholera was a disease of the slums like these in Snaithes, Yorkshire, England. In the 1850's, thousands of people died of cholera. Pioneering doctors, such as John Snow in London, proved that the disease was caused by germs in water and helped reduce the number of outbreaks of cholera.

Dirty water supplies

A clue to the cause of the cholera outbreak was found by a London doctor called John Snow. Snow was the doctor who had first introduced chloroform to Queen Victoria. He was able to show that, in one small area of London, all the victims of the disease had drunk from the same water pump. This proved that water from the pump was infected with cholera germs, so the pump was blocked, and the outbreak stopped. Snow showed how important it is to keep water supplies clean. His discovery has helped reduce the number of cholera outbreaks in many countries.

The start of a new science

Another scientist who became interested in bacteria was Robert Koch. His work started a new science, called **bacteriology**, the study of bacteria. Koch was born in 1843 in Klausthal, Germany. He studied medicine at the University of Göttingen then worked as a doctor from 1872 to 1880. He began to study bacteria using only very simple equipment such as a microscope, which made the tiny bacteria easy to see. Eventually, he found a way of growing bacteria in a dish, and he used coloured dyes to show exactly what the bacteria looked like. He also found a way of separating out one type of bacteria from a mixture of bacteria. This made it much easier to study bacteria.

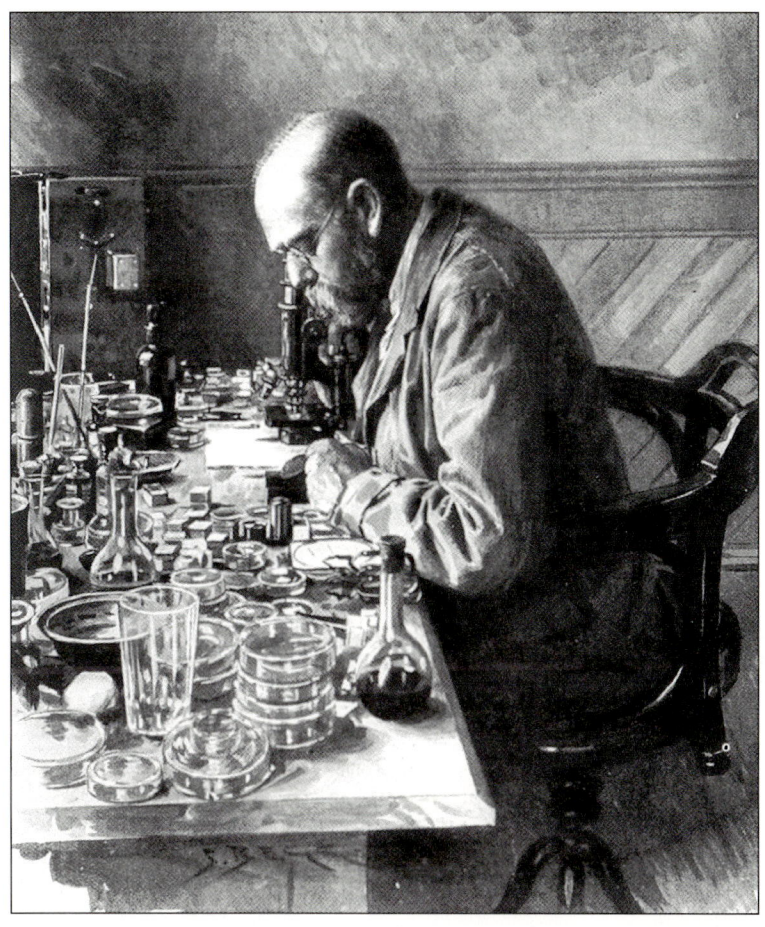

◀ **Robert Koch (1843–1910)** at work in his laboratory. He is examining a microscope slide that holds bacteria. His discovery of the germs that cause tuberculosis and cholera made it much easier to detect these diseases.

▼ **The cholera germ**. This picture of the cholera bacterium or germ, magnified about 9000 times, was produced using a powerful modern microscope. Robert Koch invented the techniques of growing and colouring bacteria so that they could be seen more easily under a microscope. This helped scientists to study bacteria and produce cures to many diseases.

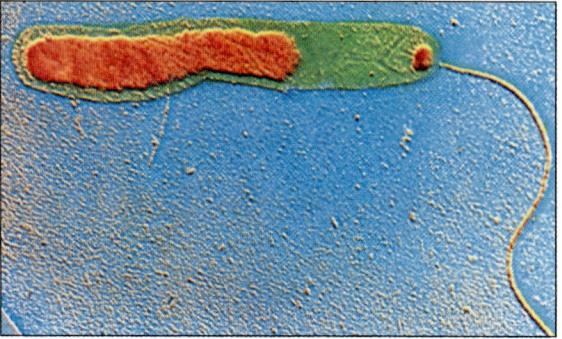

In 1882 Koch discovered the bacteria that cause tuberculosis. In 1876, he discovered the life cycle of the bacteria causing anthrax, a disease of cattle and sheep. In 1884, he travelled to Egypt to study cholera, and discovered the cholera bacteria. When he returned to Germany, he was made a professor of medicine at the University of Berlin. He was awarded the **Nobel Prize** for Medicine in 1905.

Robert Koch died in 1910. Although he did not discover the cure for tuberculosis or cholera he made it easier for other scientists to study the bacteria that cause these diseases and this, in turn, made it easier to find a cure. In 1906 a vaccine against the tuberculosis germ was discovered and people can now be protected against the disease.

The lady with the lamp

When Florence Nightingale told her parents in 1843 that she wanted to become a nurse, they were horrified. Florence's family was quite wealthy and in those days, nursing was not a job for a respectable girl. Nurses were mostly untrained and ignorant. They slept on duty and were often drunk. It is because of the work of Florence Nightingale that nursing is a respected profession today.

Florence began by attending a school for nurses in Germany because, at the time, this was the only place that gave nurses a proper training. When she had finished her training, she returned to London where she got a job running a hospital for sick women.

Appalling conditions

In 1853 war broke out between Britain, France, Turkey and Sardinia, and Russia. The fighting in the Crimea, a small piece of land jutting out into the Black Sea, went on for months. Stories reached Britain of the terrible hardships suffered by the wounded soldiers in the poor hospitals at the battle front. The British government sent Florence, with 38 other nurses, to help care for them.

When they arrived at the town of Scutari, Florence and her nurses found conditions worse than expected. There was no soap, no towels and no clothes. The wounded soldiers were lying in their uniforms, covered in blood. Rats infested the filthy hospital, and the smell of the toilets blew into the corridors and wards.

After much opposition from the distrustful army doctors Florence and her nurses set to work. They soon had the wards clean and in good order. They set up a laundry and fed the men good food. Florence nagged the army commander until proper toilets were installed. The hospital became a cleaner and safer place and each night Florence would walk through the wards carrying a light to check that all was well. She became known as the 'Lady with the Lamp'.

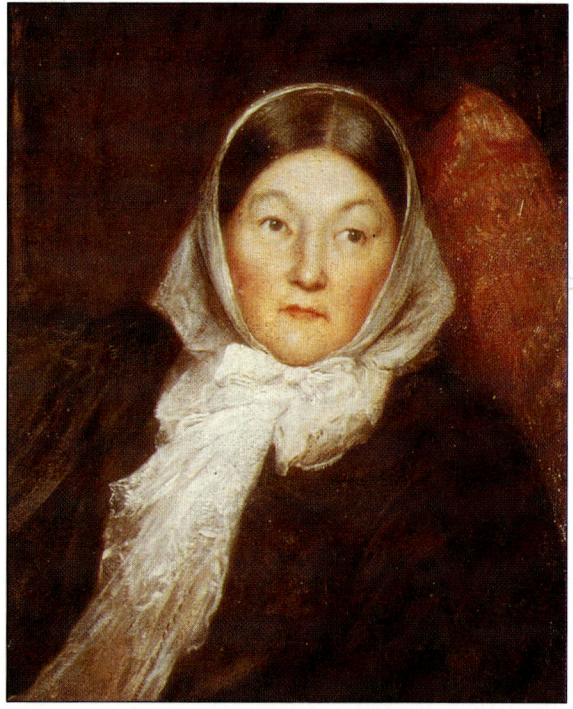

Florence Nightingale (1820–1910). She showed that nurses could be very helpful to doctors and patients. Her work in the Crimea saved many lives and led to the setting up of proper training schools for nurses.

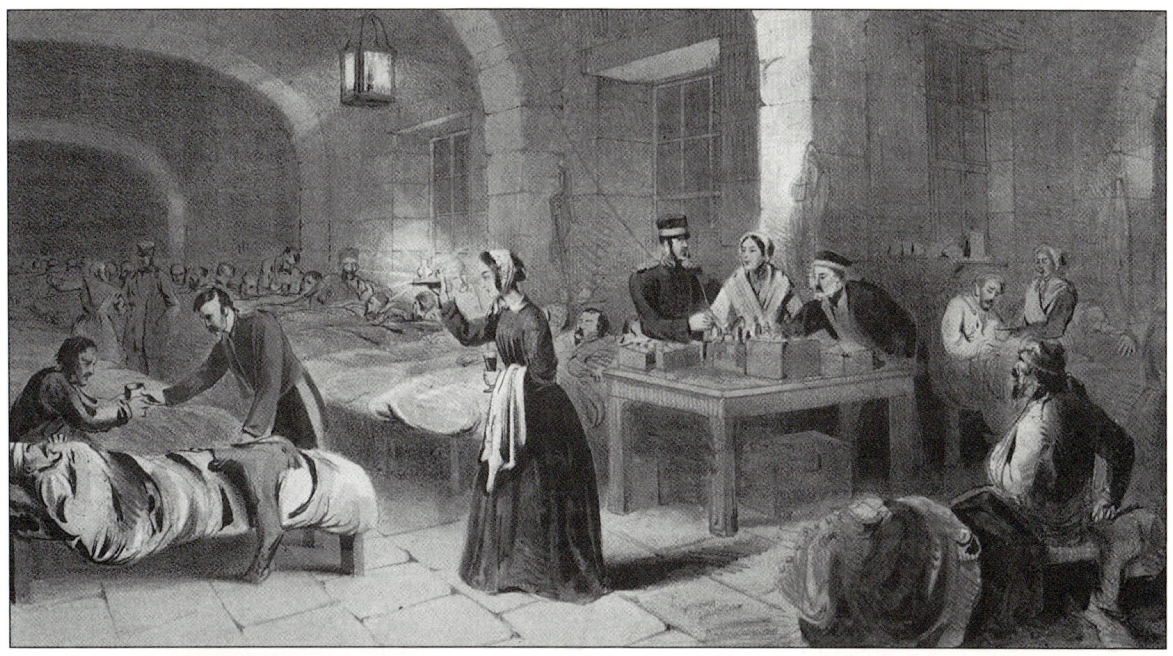

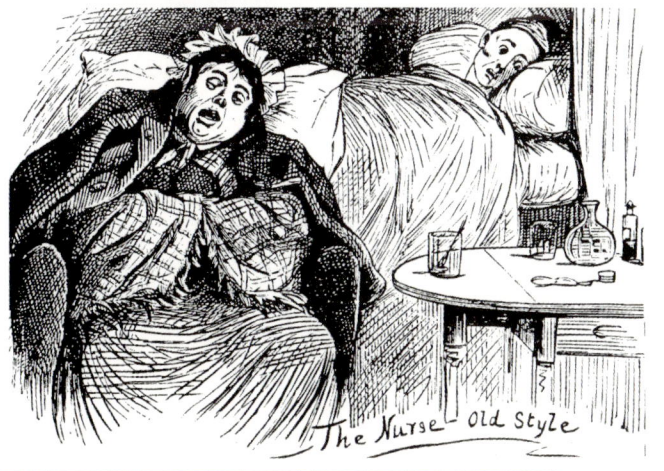

▲ **Florence Nightingale in the military hospital** shown with a lamp, checking that all is well with the patients at Scutari. Known as the 'Lady with the Lamp', Florence insisted that hospital wards should be clean and airy as shown. Before her work, hospitals were often dark, smelly and dirty.

◀ **The nurse – old style**. Before Florence Nightingale, nurses did not take good care of their patients. They were often asleep, drunk on duty, or stole from their patients. Thanks to Florence's work, nurses are now properly trained.

A school for nurses

When Florence returned to Britain, grateful people collected a large sum of money for her. In 1860 she used this to start a school for nurses at St Thomas's Hospital in London. Training at the school was strict. Nurses had to live at the hospital, they were not allowed to leave the hospital alone and they had to keep a diary, which was inspected each month. Of course, they also received the very best training in nursing and medicine. Other schools were soon started and the number of trained nurses increased. For the rest of her life, Florence worked to improve the standard of nursing. When she died in 1910, nurses had become important and respected members of every hospital.

The first woman doctor

For most of the history of medicine, all doctors were men. Why was this? Some people said it was because women did not have the strength to carry out operations. This strange idea was proved wrong by Elizabeth Blackwell. Despite a hard struggle, she became the first woman doctor in the United States and Britain.

A solitary student

Elizabeth was born in Bristol, in England, in 1821 but her family moved to the United States in 1832. Elizabeth's parents were caring people. They gave their children a good education and they supported many good causes, such as the fight against slavery in the United States. When Elizabeth decided she wanted to become a doctor, they supported her even though the idea must have surprised them at first.

At the time, there were no women doctors and no medical school would let Elizabeth attend classes. So Elizabeth studied on her own, using the few medical books she could find. After her father died in 1838, Elizabeth worked during the day to support the family of nine children. She continued her lonely medical studies in the evenings.

Top of the class

Eventually, Elizabeth found a small medical school called Geneva Medical College, in New York State, that would

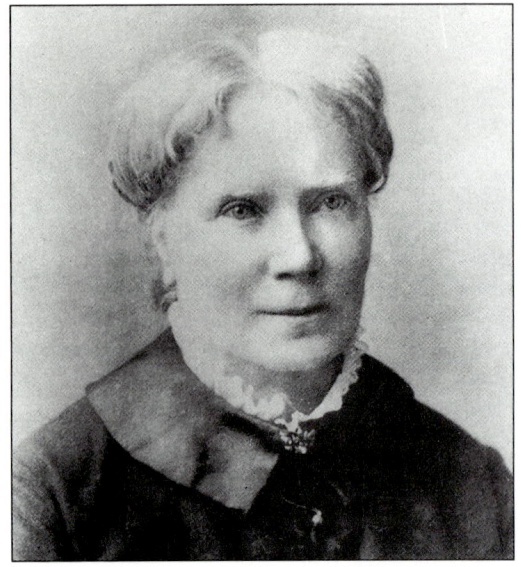

Elizabeth Blackwell (1821–1910) was the first woman doctor in the United States and Britain. She started schools where women could study medicine and proved that women could be good doctors.

accept her as a student. She studied hard and earned the respect of her teachers and fellow students. In 1849 she finished her studies and came first in her class.

Elizabeth Blackwell was the first woman to qualify as a doctor anywhere in the world. She completed her education in Europe. She studied in Paris and at Saint Bartholomew's Hospital in London, where she gained valuable experience.

Opportunities for other women

Elizabeth then returned to the United States. She began work as a doctor in New York City. As well as her paying patients, Elizabeth helped the poor of the

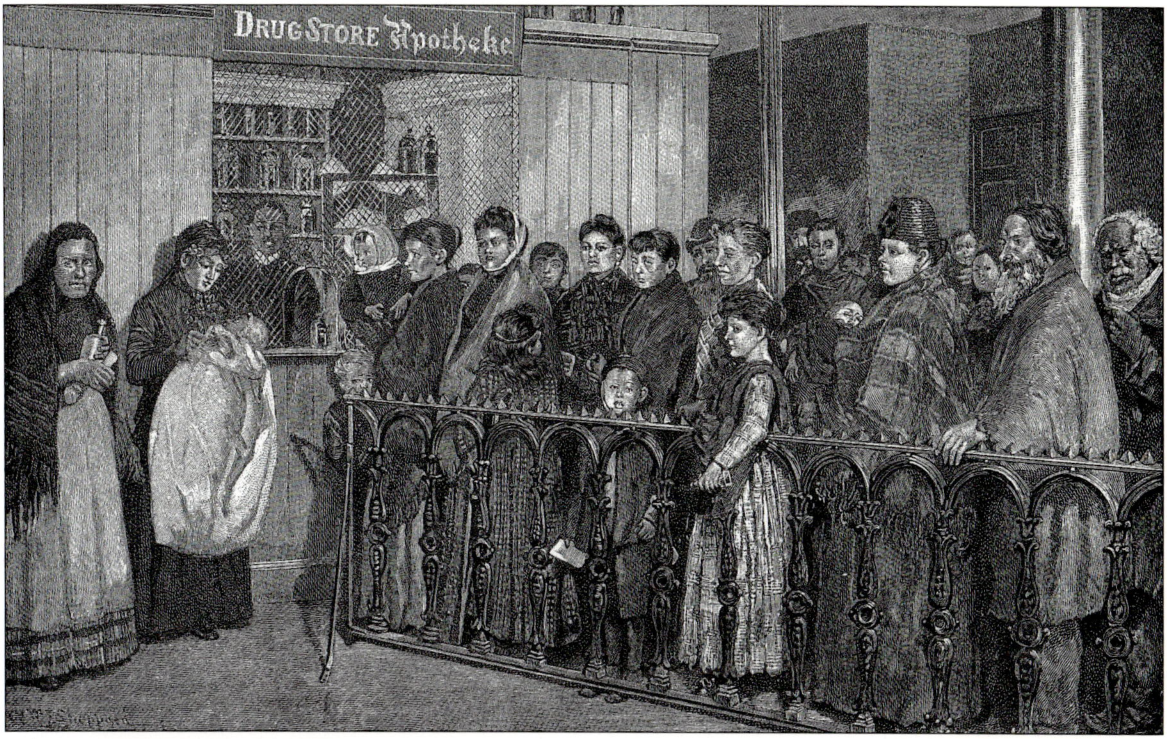

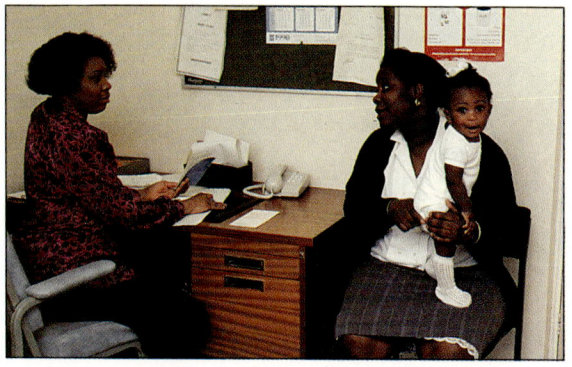

Elizabeth Blackwell's hospital in New York in the late 1800s. Some doctors, such as Elizabeth Blackwell, provided free drugs and treatment for the poor.

city by providing medicines free of charge. In 1857 she opened a hospital called the New York Infirmary for Women and Children. Eleven years later, the hospital became a medical school where women could train to become doctors. At this time, other medical schools in the United States were also starting to let women study medicine.

Elizabeth returned to England determined to help British women become doctors. In 1869 she became the first woman doctor to be allowed to practise medicine in Britain. In 1874 she helped to start a medical school for women in London. It was called the London School of Medicine for Women.

A woman doctor at work. Elizabeth Blackwell helped to show that women could be good doctors.

As a result of her work, medical schools in Britain began to let women study medicine. When she died in 1910, no one doubted that women could be good doctors.

The new surgery

The discovery of pain-killing substances, such as chloroform, made surgical operations less painful but surgery was still dangerous. In 1860 in Glasgow, Scotland, nearly half of the patients who had operations died soon afterwards. Their wounds became infected and their blood would become poisoned. Despite Pasteur's discovery that tiny germs were carried in the air, most doctors thought that a poisonous gas in the air caused disease. They did not think it was important to wear clean clothes and continued to do

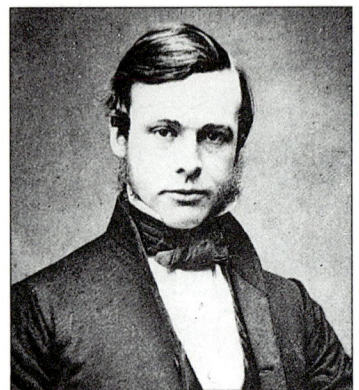

Joseph Lister (1827–1912), the English surgeon who pioneered antiseptic techniques in surgery. This picture was made when he was in his late twenties.

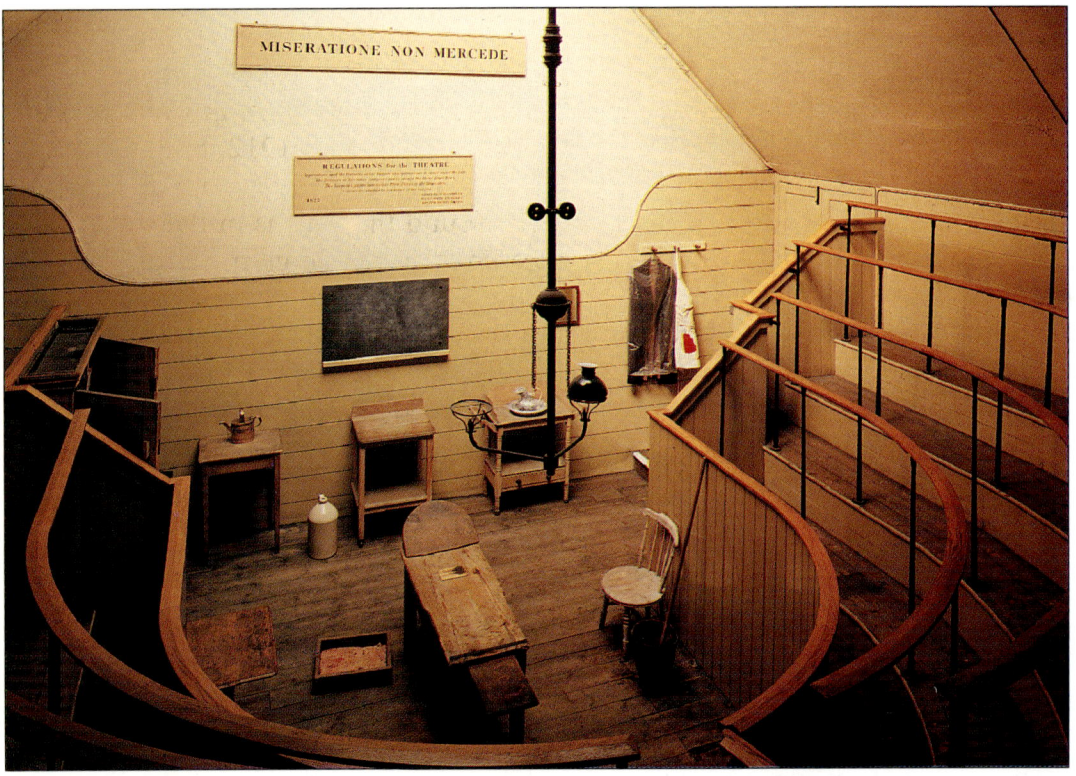

An operating theatre at the time of Lister built in 1821 at Saint Thomas's Hospital, London. The bare boards, rows of seats for onlookers, and the surgeon's bloodstained apron hanging on the wall, show that the theatre could not have been hygienic.

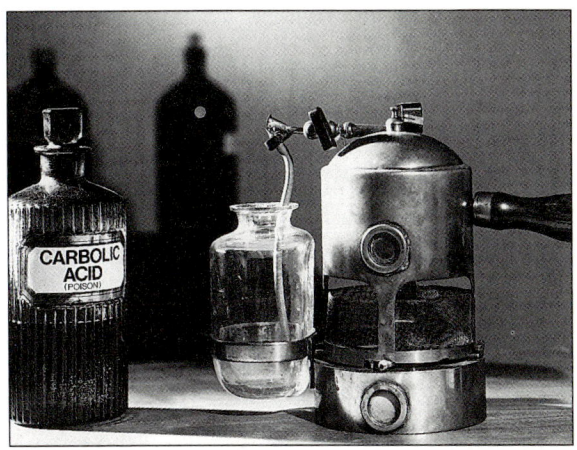

Lister's carbolic spray. This spray was used by Lister to fill the air with fine droplets of carbolic acid. The spray killed any germs in the air.

operations in dirty coats stained with blood and covered with pus. Some patients thought that the dirtier a doctor's coat the better. A dirty coat showed that the doctor had done many operations and so must be an expert!

Joseph Lister's liquid

In 1865 an English surgeon called Joseph Lister was working in Glasgow. He read about Pasteur's discoveries and wondered if tiny germs, like those that caused wine to go bad, might also be the cause of infections in wounds. Lister had heard of an **antiseptic**, or germ-killing substance, called carbolic acid. This had been used for cleaning sewers. He decided to use carbolic acid to wash his hands and instruments in before performing an operation. He also soaked bandages in carbolic acid. In 1875 he made a small machine that sprayed carbolic acid into the air. This was used during operations, and killed germs in the air.

Lister's methods were successful and the number of deaths following his operations dropped. However, many surgeons refused to use his methods because they complained that it took too long to wash everything. One famous surgeon made a joke of Lister's ideas. He told his students as they entered the room, 'Shut the door quickly or one of Mister Lister's germs may come in.' Gradually, however, Lister's ideas were accepted, and surgery became much safer.

Keeping germs out

Lister was given many honours. In 1877 he became Professor of Surgery at King's College Hospital in London. By the time he died in 1912, his methods had been developed even further. It had been found that germs in the air were less important than germs in clothing and on hands. The carbolic spray dropped out of use.

Instead of antiseptic surgery, in which germs are killed by antiseptics, surgeons began using **aseptic** methods. These new methods tried to stop germs entering the operating room, or theatre, in the first place. The theatre is kept completely clean and germs are removed from the air before it enters the theatre. Surgeons wear masks and rubber gloves. This means that germs in their breath and on their skin cannot reach the patient. These methods are used today, and make modern surgery safer and more successful.

The fight against malaria

I f you have ever been bitten by a mosquito, you know how uncomfortable it can be. Some mosquitos, however, do more than give an itchy bite. They also carry a common disease called **malaria**. Malaria is a disease found in tropical countries that produces a high fever. It is caused by very small animals that enter the bloodstream and live inside the body. These animals, called **parasites**, are carried around by a type of mosquito and they get into the body when the mosquito punctures the skin. The person who discovered how mosquitoes carry malaria was a British doctor called Patrick Manson.

Research in the Far East

Patrick Manson was born in 1844. He studied medicine at Aberdeen in Scotland where he learned a lot about parasites, the little animals or plants that live in or feed on other animals or plants. Manson then went to China and spent 24 years studying the diseases found there. He started a medical school in Hong Kong, which later became the University of Hong Kong. Manson also

Patrick Manson (1844–1922), the Scottish doctor who showed that insects are responsible for spreading diseases such as malaria and elephantiasis. His work on malaria earned him the nickname, 'Mosquito Manson'.

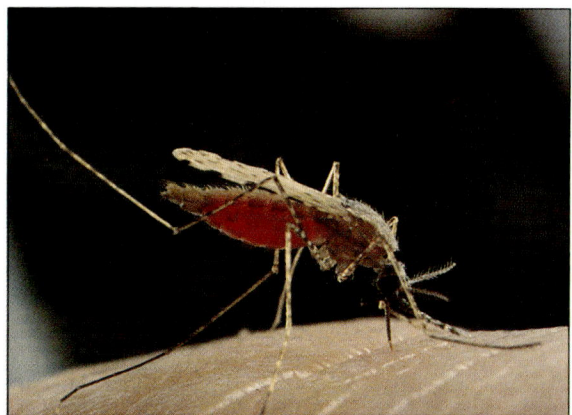

The female Anopheles mosquito which carries the malaria parasite. When the mosquito bites a victim in order to feed on some blood, she injects a liquid into the wound to stop the blood drying up. This liquid contains the parasite that causes the disease, malaria.

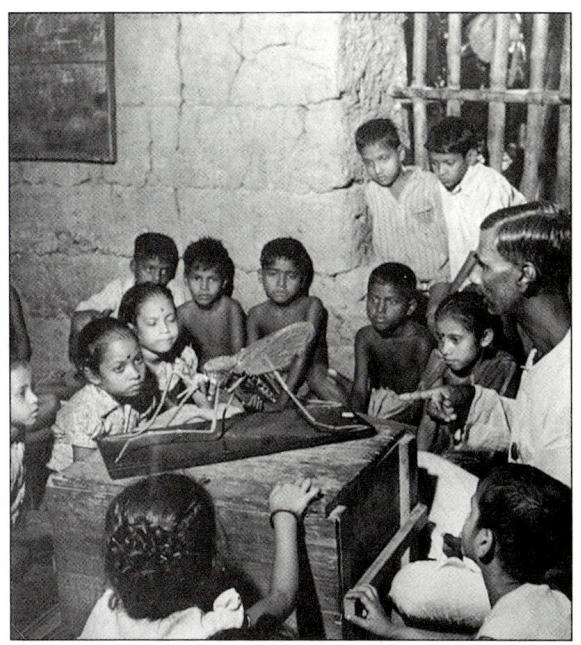

Malaria today. Malaria is still common in countries like India. These children are learning about the mosquito that carries the disease and how to protect themselves from it.

founded the famous London School of Tropical Medicine in England.

Manson was the first person to prove that some parasites could be carried by insects. He discovered that a disease called elephantiasis is caused by worms carried in the stomachs of mosquitoes. The worms block the channels that carry liquids around the body and this makes parts of the body swell up.

Solving the malaria mystery

In 1894 Manson met in London a doctor called Ronald Ross who was in the Indian Medical Service. Manson suggested that malaria might also be caused by parasites carried by mosquitoes. Ross decided that in India,

where malaria was common, he would look for the malaria-carrying mosquitoes. In 1897, Ross found the type of mosquito that carried the malaria parasites.

However, Manson wanted better proof. He sent two of his assistants to live in the swamps near Rome in Italy. The people living near these swamps often caught malaria but they thought it was because of the poisonous gases from the swamp. Manson's assistants avoided the mosquitoes and slept at night in a mosquito-proof hut. They did not get malaria and this showed that the disease was not caused by poisonous gases found in the swamp.

Wiping out the mosquitoes

Manson did another experiment. He allowed mosquitoes that had fed on the blood of malaria sufferers to bite two volunteers who had never been abroad in their lives. Both volunteers caught the disease. This proved that the disease was carried by the mosquito and was passed on when the mosquito bit someone.

Manson's experiments showed what had to be done to eradicate, or get rid of, malaria. The mosquitoes had to be removed. Insecticides were sprayed on places where the mosquitoes bred. Mosquito-repellent creams, mosquito-proof clothes and nets were invented. Effective drugs were also developed. The disease is still common in parts of Africa, South America and Asia but Manson's dedicated work did a great deal to help prevent and control it.

Blood replacement

I f you have an accident, or cut yourself, you might bleed a lot. You might even need to be given some extra blood to make up for the blood you have lost. Giving a person blood from another person is called **blood transfusion**. Blood transfusions save lives. People often need transfusions after serious accidents or when they are undergoing surgery. Transfusions are also given to people suffering from some blood diseases.

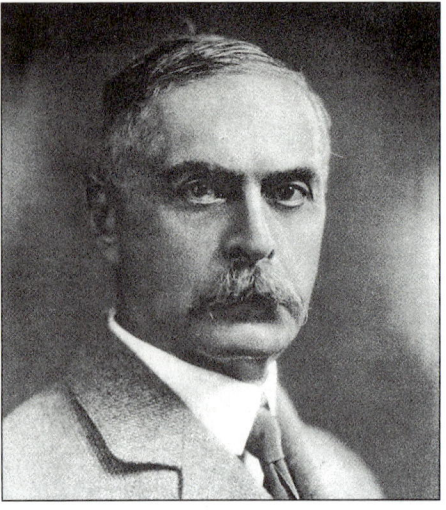

Karl Landsteiner (1868–1943) discovered that there are four major blood groups. This discovery was essential for the safe use of blood transfusions.

Blood is not always the same

Different people have different types of blood. These different types of blood are called **blood groups**. During a transfusion, a person must only be given blood of the right type, or group, so very careful checks must be made before blood from one person can be given to another.

Over 500 years ago, the Incas of South America were successfully carrying out blood transfusions without knowing about blood groups. This was possible because most South American indians have blood of the same group. This meant that they could safely give transfusions without testing the blood.

Elsewhere blood transfusions were not successful. In 1628 an Italian called Giovanni Colle attempted to give blood to sick people. Most of his patients died because they received blood from the wrong group and, as a result, blood transfusions were made illegal.

Discovering blood groups

The fact that there are different blood groups was discovered in 1909 by an Austrian doctor called Karl Landsteiner. He found that there are four groups of blood, which he called types A, B, AB, and O. The differences between the types of blood can only be seen under a microscope, and by using chemical tests. Landsteiner's discovery meant that, at last, it was possible to give the correct type of blood to a person needing a transfusion. In 1930 Landsteiner was awarded the Nobel Prize for Medicine for his discovery.

In 1922 Landsteiner moved from Vienna to the United States. He continued to study blood and, in 1940, made another discovery. He found that

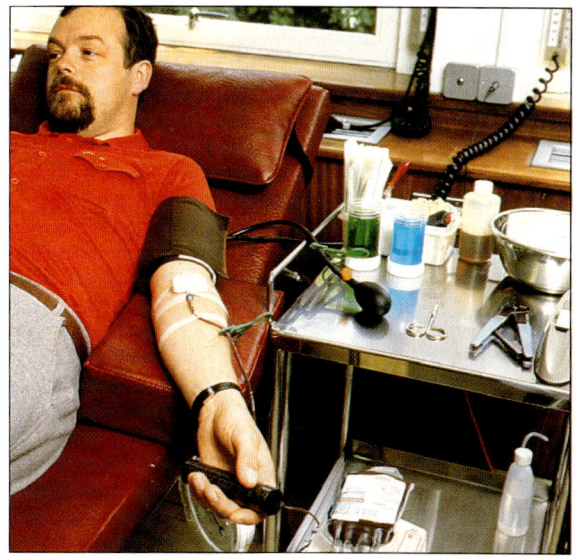

blood was more complicated than he had first thought. He noticed that some people who had received the correct type of blood in a transfusion did not make a good recovery. Eventually, Landsteiner found that this was because some people had a substance called the **rhesus factor** in their blood. This had to be taken into account when blood was given to these people. It was also found that sometimes a baby without the rhesus factor in its blood could be born ill. To avoid this, these babies are given a transfusion of new, safe blood soon after birth.

▲ **Giving blood**. People either give or sell their blood to hospitals. The blood is taken from the arm through a thin tube and is then stored in refrigerated 'blood banks' until needed.

▶ **Testing blood**. All blood must be carefully checked to make sure that it does not contain any dangerous germs. The technician on the left is checking that the blood sample is free from the antibodies found in AIDS sufferers.

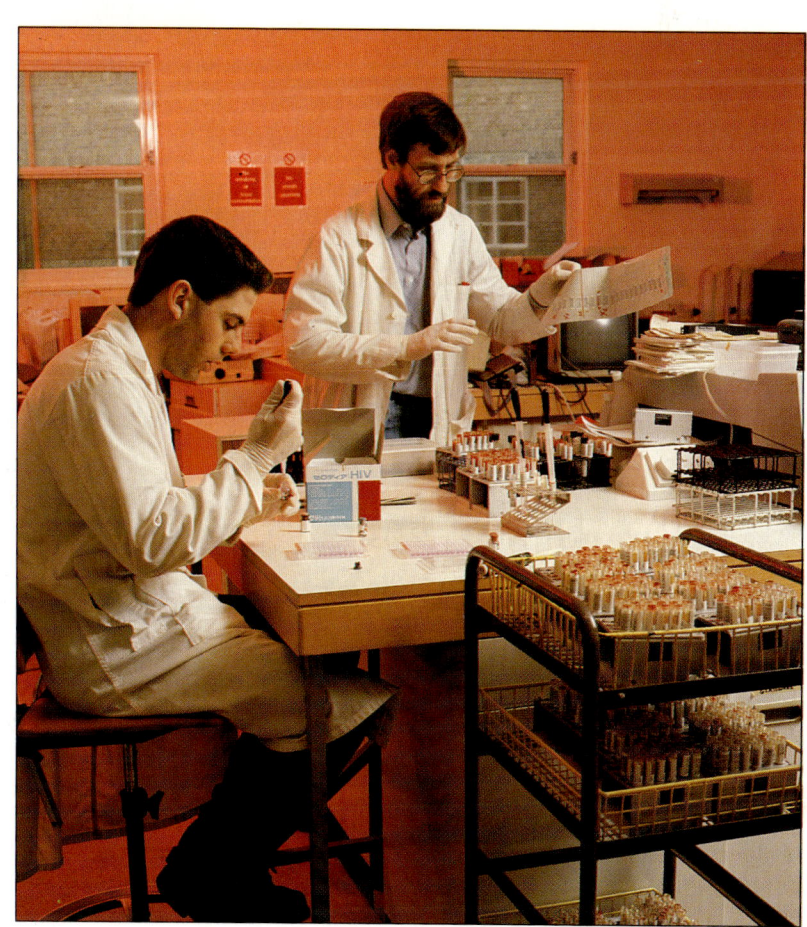

Magic bullets

What do you do if you have a sore throat or a headache? You probably take a pill, such as aspirin, to make the pain go away. Drugs like this are used every day, but they have not always been available. The drugs used in ancient times were made mainly from plants and herbs but they did not always work well. Although they sometimes reduced pain, these early drugs did not kill the germs or bacteria that caused diseases. The first drug that killed bacteria was developed in 1910 by Paul Ehrlich.

The colourful world of bacteria

Paul Ehrlich was a German scientist who was born in 1854. He studied medicine and became a teacher of medicine in Berlin in 1887. In 1890 he went to work in Robert Koch's laboratory. Koch was studying bacteria, and he had discovered that certain coloured dyes would stick to bacteria, making them easy to see with a microscope.

Paul Ehrlich tried out different dyes to see which bacteria particular colours would stick to. By using dyes, he

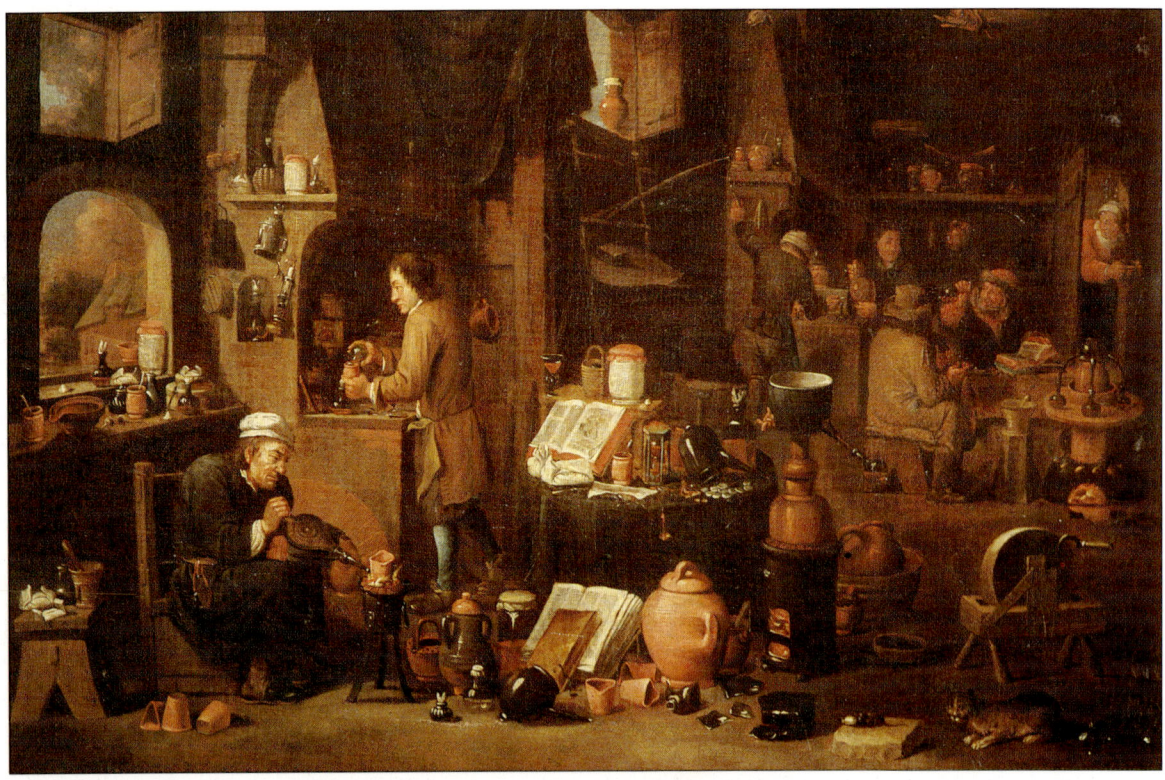

A doctor's shop in the 1600s. The doctor mixes simple drugs made from plants and minerals following a recipe in the open book by his side. His assistant uses bellows to blow a fire which heats another potion. In the background, a customer peeps cautiously round the door.

34

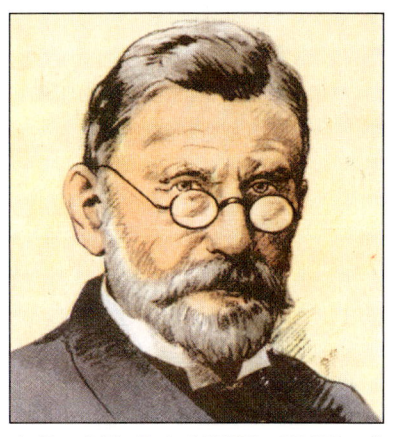

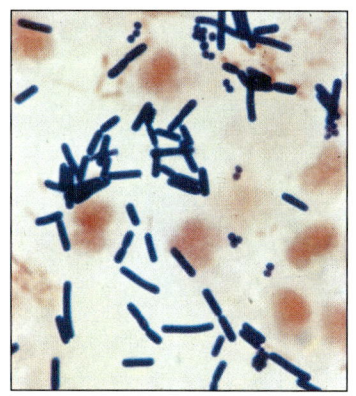

▲ **Germs from an infected cut**. This photograph, enlarged about 1000 times, shows germs (blue-black dots) which cause wounds to rot, but the red blobs are harmless bacteria. Ehrlich mixed drugs with the dyes that stuck to germs and the drugs then killed the germs.

▲ **Paul Ehrlich (1854–1915)**, discovered the first drug that could destroy germs inside the body. He showed that drugs could cure disease without harming the patient and was awarded the Nobel Prize for Medicine in 1908.

discovered that blood contains substances called antibodies that kill germs entering the body. This discovery helped doctors to understand why vaccination worked. A vaccine causes the body to produce antibodies that are specially designed to kill certain germs. Paul Ehrlich was awarded the Nobel Prize for Medicine in 1908 for his work on antibodies.

Aiming at individual germs

Paul Ehrlich dreamed of finding a chemical that would kill harmful germs without hurting the healthy parts of the body. He called these substances 'magic bullets' because they would seek out and kill the harmful germs. He first discovered a red dye that attacked the bacteria that causes sleeping sickness, a disease found in Africa. Next he tried to find a cure for **syphilis**, a disease that causes swellings and rashes and

eventually affects the brain. The problem was not to find a drug that killed the syphilis germ. Doctors knew that mercury killed the germ but, unfortunately, mercury also poisoned the patient! Ehrlich wanted a drug that only killed the germs.

The answer was to combine a poison with a dye that stuck only to the syphilis germs. Ehrlich tried many different combinations of poisons and dyes. Eventually, in 1910, after testing over 600 different combinations, he found one that worked. The drug, called preparation 606, was the first effective treatment for syphilis.

Ehrlich's discovery made it possible for other doctors to find ways of producing drugs to fight many more diseases. In 1932 a German called Gerhard Domagk invented a drug to cure scarlet fever. This was the first of an important type of drug, called **sulpha drugs**, that could cure illnesses such as **meningitis**, a serious brain disease. Many of these diseases were major killers of young children. The development of drugs has meant that few people today die from such illnesses.

The wonder drug

If you have tonsillitis, your doctor might give you a drug called **penicillin** to kill the bacteria causing the pain. Drugs like penicillin are called **antibiotics**. The word 'antibiotic' comes from two Greek words meaning 'against' and 'life'. Penicillin was discovered by a Scottish doctor called Alexander Fleming.

A wartime doctor

Alexander Fleming was born in 1881 in Ayrshire, in Scotland. He studied medicine at Saint Mary's Hospital Medical School in London and he specialized in the study of bacteria. During the First World War, he served as a doctor with the British army. During the war, he saw that thousands of soldiers died after small cuts became infected by bacteria. There was, at this time, no drug to kill the bacteria causing the infections. In 1918 when the war ended, Fleming returned to Saint Mary's Hospital to teach and to study the bacteria that infected wounds.

A lucky accident

In his experiments, Fleming used small, flat dishes containing a jelly-like substance. Bacteria were allowed to grow in these dishes, so that they could be studied. One day in 1928 Fleming noticed that some mould was growing in one of the dishes. It was like the mould which grows on stale bread. The mould must have blown in through the open window. At first, Fleming was annoyed and thought that the experiment was ruined.

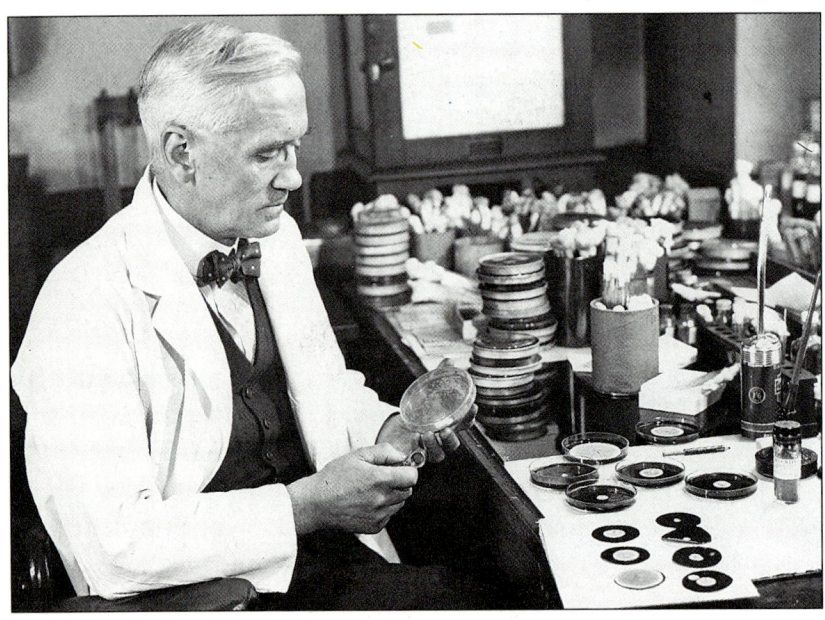

Alexander Fleming (1881–1955), discoverer of the wonder drug penicillin, examining a small dish used to grow bacteria for his experiments. Fleming discovered penicillin when a tiny piece of mould blew in through the window and ruined one of his experiments. But he quickly saw that the mould could be used to kill bacteria.

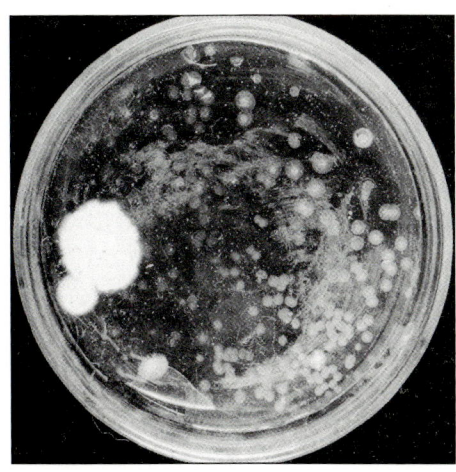

Fleming's dish of penicillin mould. The mould on the left has killed most of the bacteria growing near it. To the right of the dish bacteria still grows. This was the clue that led Fleming to discover the first antibiotic drug.

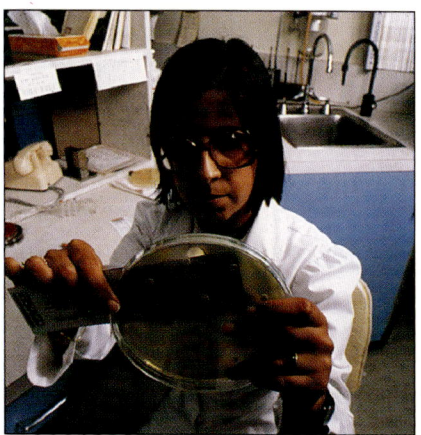

Discovering new antibiotics. Today new antibiotics have been developed to treat diseases that penicillin does not cure. This researcher is studying the germ-killing action of a mould in a flat dish. The discoloured area around the white mould is where bacteria have been destroyed by the mould.

However, when he took a closer look, Fleming saw that all the bacteria around the mould were dead. The mould was producing something that killed the bacteria. He grew more of this mould, which was called *penicillium notatum,* and he found that the mould could kill many different bacteria. Fleming then extracted the substance that was so deadly to bacteria from the mould. He called this new bacteria-killing substance penicillin. More experiments showed that penicillin could be used to treat diseases caused by bacteria. However, Fleming could not find a way to make large quantities of penicillin.

Mass-produced penicillin

Twelve years later, in 1940, an Australian professor called Howard Florey, and a young German chemist called Ernst Chain, found a way of making penicillin in quantity. They tested the drug thoroughly using white mice. The tests were successful and the drug went into production. It was just in time to save the lives of many soldiers wounded in the Second World War. Penicillin became known as the 'wonder drug' because it attacked many different kinds of bacteria.

Alexander Fleming, Howard Florey and Ernst Chain were awarded the Nobel Prize for Medicine in 1945 for their discoveries. They led the way for other scientists to develop many other antibiotics. These are very important, because penicillin does not kill every bacteria and, also, some people are allergic to penicillin. This means they cannot be given it as a treatment. Without alternative antibiotics, these people would become very ill and many would probably die.

Healing the sick mind

Not all illnesses are caused by germs and bacteria. Some illnesses are called **mental illnesses** because they affect the mind. In the past, people with mental illnesses were often treated very badly. They were sometimes thought to have evil spirits inside their heads. In the Bethlehem Hospital, nicknamed 'Bedlam', in London, England, patients were chained to the walls to stop them doing damage. Other patients were kept locked in boxes with only their head poking out of the top.

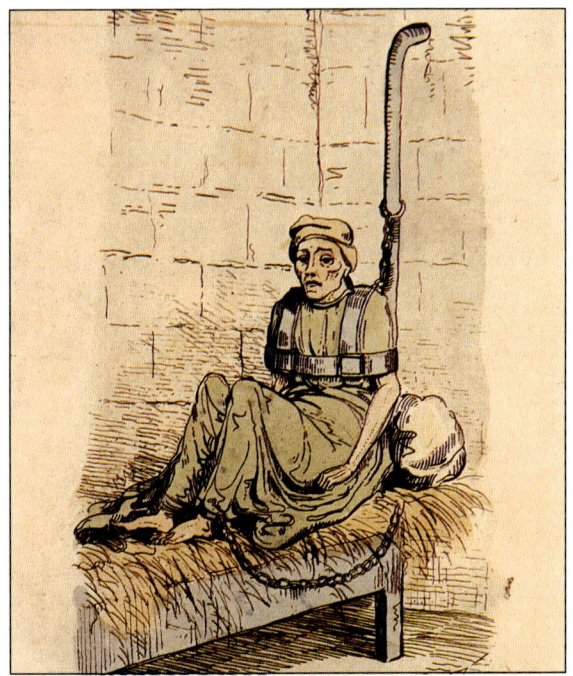

A patient in the 'Bedlam' hospital in London in about 1800 chained to the wall and shackled to stop him doing damage. This terrible treatment of mental patients continued until Freud showed that such patients were not evil or possessed by spirits.

Today, people with mental illness are treated with kindness. They are given drugs to calm them and doctors talk to them, so that they can understand their problems. Many patients are treated using methods worked out by a doctor called Sigmund Freud.

Sigmund Freud

Sigmund Freud was born in 1856 in Freiberg, Czechoslovakia. In 1859 the Freud family moved to Vienna, the capital of Austria. The family was poor but they managed to save enough money to allow young Sigmund to study medicine. In 1882 Freud began to work with another doctor called Josef Breuer who treated mentally ill patients using a new method. Breuer would gently persuade his patient to go to sleep. He would then talk to the lightly sleeping patient, and discuss their illness with them. Sometimes, this helped the patient get better. Sometimes patients got better if they were simply allowed to talk about how they felt. This interested Freud and he began to study the way the human mind works.

The hidden mind

Freud gradually realized that people keep many thoughts and feelings hidden in their mind. Bad memories and feelings are buried deep and often cannot be remembered. Although these memories and feelings are hidden, they may affect the patient's health. Freud developed a way of finding these hidden memories. The patient would lie on a couch and talk about anything they wanted to. As the patient talked, painful feelings or long-forgotten memories were sometimes revealed. The patient was then encouraged to think about, or analyse, the worries that were making them ill. This process is called **psychoanalysis**, which means studying the mind. Freud was also interested in people's dreams. He thought that these revealed hidden desires and memories.

Many other doctors came to Vienna to learn about Freud's ideas. When he died in London in 1939, the importance of his work was well known. Today, however, some of his ideas are thought to be wrong. Doctors now realize that not all mental problems are caused by forgotten memories and they use drugs to cure some mental illnesses. However, Freud's new approach to the problems of mentally-ill patients did lead to a more sympathetic attitude and psychoanalysis is still used to treat some cases of mental illness.

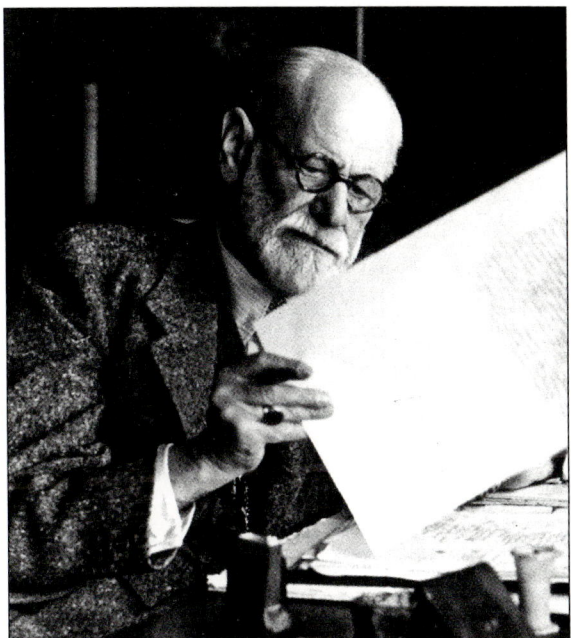

▲ **Sigmund Freud (1856–1939)**, explorer of the unconscious mind. Freud found ways of revealing feelings hidden deep within the mind. Patients often became better when they talked about these feelings.

▶ **A dream of drowning**. Freud believed that our unconscious feelings are revealed in our dreams. By studying his own dreams and those of his patients, Freud decided that in our dreams there were signs, or symbols, of our feelings. A dream of drowning may reveal feelings of helplessness and despair.

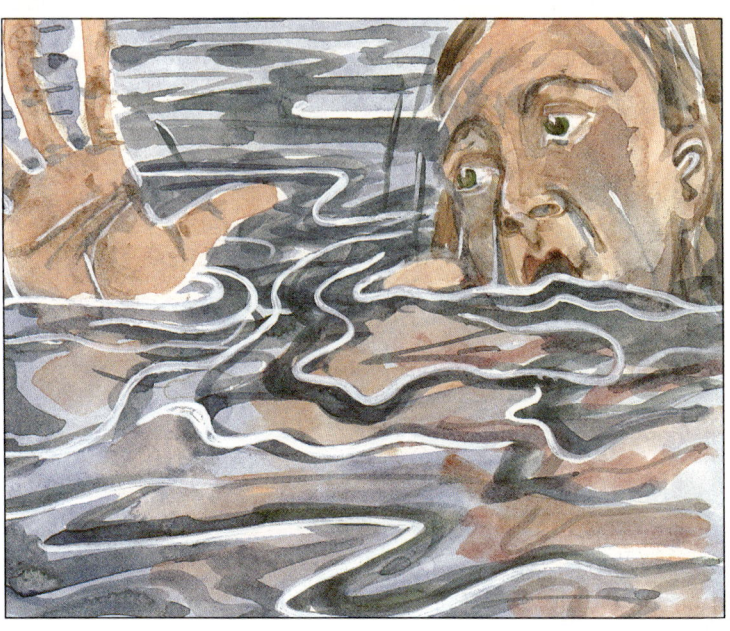

Fighting paralysis

Not long ago, **polio**, or poliomyelitis, was a feared disease. Polio affects mostly young children and it often paralyses them so that they cannot move or walk. Sometimes, polio sufferers have trouble breathing. In the past, they had to spend long times in a machine, called an iron lung, that helped them to breathe. Many people died from polio and many others were crippled by it. A young American doctor called Jonas Salk set out to find a vaccine to protect people from the disease.

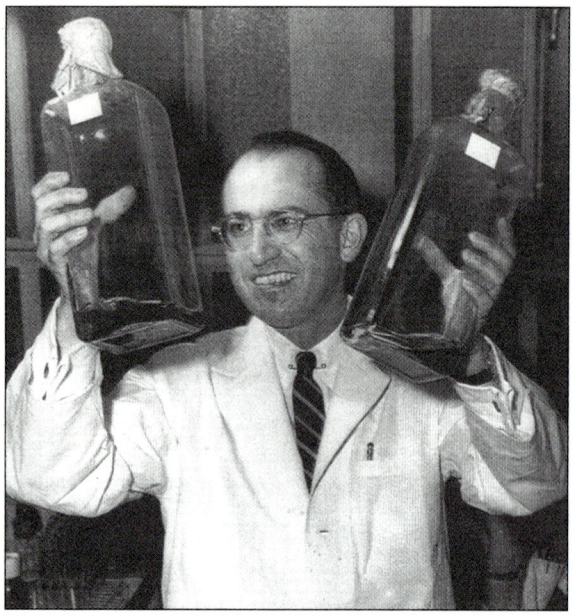

Jonas Salk (1914–), developed a vaccine which prevented polio in 1954. Now polio is practically unknown in many countries.

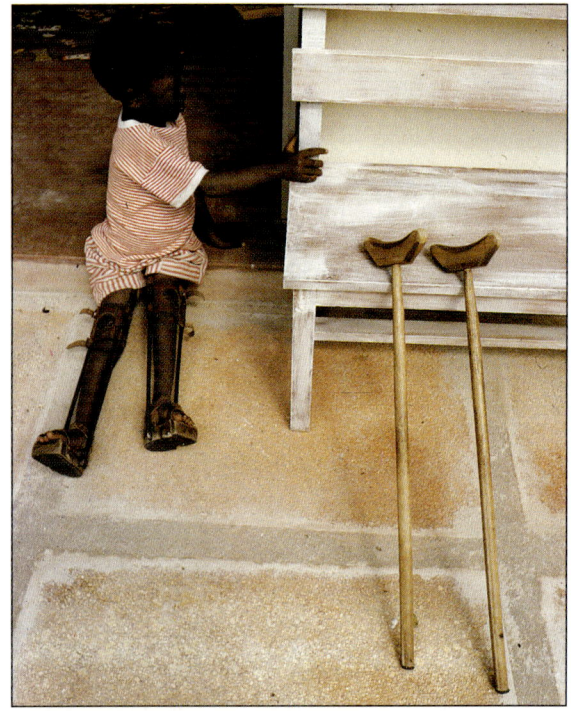

Polio, a childhood disease, which crippled and killed many children in the past. This polio sufferer has steel braces on his legs to strengthen them, and crutches to help get around.

The price of success

Jonas Salk was born in New York in 1914. He was a brilliant student and studied medicine at the New York College of Medicine. In 1947 he began to study **viruses**. These are extremely small particles that cause disease. They are smaller than bacteria, and live inside plants and animals. Even though they are small, viruses cause many diseases. Influenza, the common cold, measles and mumps are all caused by viruses. So is polio. However, there are hundreds of different viruses that cause polio and this made it very difficult for Jonas Salk to produce a vaccine.

It took Salk three years to identify

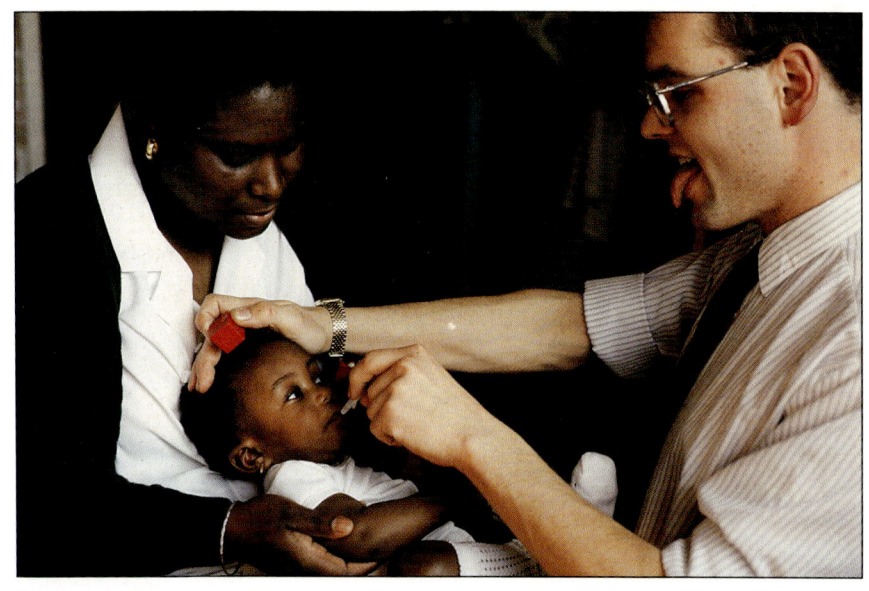

Taking polio vaccine. There is no need to be frightened of an injection. Polio vaccine is swallowed and, in a second, you are safe from polio.

most of the polio viruses. He found that there were three main types of virus causing polio. Any vaccine would have to work against all three types. His experiments were also very expensive. They cost over a million dollars. He also used over 30 000 monkeys in his experiments to try out the different vaccines. At last, in 1953, he succeeded. A vaccine was produced and tested on 1000 children and adults in Pittsburgh in the United States. These tests showed that the vaccine worked and doctors began giving the vaccine to all children.

Medicine in a sugar lump

At first, quite a large number of children who had been injected with the Salk vaccine still caught polio. For a brief time it looked as if all the work had been wasted. Perhaps the vaccine did not work. However, it was discovered that some vaccine had been made incorrectly.

When properly made vaccine was used, it was effective. By 1960 there were few cases of polio in the United States and other countries where the vaccine was used. Salk's vaccine had saved the lives of thousands of children and had prevented many more from becoming crippled.

In the 1960s Salk's vaccine was replaced by a vaccine discovered by a Russian-born doctor called Albert Sabin. Sabin came to America in 1930 and worked at the University of Cincinnati. His vaccine was more effective and was easier to give to children. Sabin's vaccine did not need to be injected using a needle but could be put on a sugar lump and swallowed. Children are no longer frightened of having an injection and are happy to swallow a lump of sugar. This means that very few children escape being treated against polio except in some poorer countries and, as a result, the disease is very rarely found.

New parts for old

Today, surgery is so advanced that it is even possible to replace unhealthy parts of the body with parts from another person. The unhealthy organ is removed from the patient and a new one put in its place by the surgeon. These operations are called **transplant operations**. The new organ usually comes from a person who has just died, perhaps in a traffic accident. One problem with transplant surgery is that the new organ sometimes does not grow successfully. This is called rejection, because the patient's body throws off, or rejects, the new organ. However, doctors have discovered drugs that prevent the rejection of new organs.

The first transplant

The first successful transplant was carried out in 1954 by an American surgeon called Joseph Murray. A patient with kidney disease was given a new kidney. The kidneys are organs that control the amount of water in the body and take waste substances out of the blood. If the kidney does not work properly, the blood becomes poisoned and the patient will die.

Kidney transplants are now a common way of treating serious kidney disease. If a transplanted kidney is rejected by the patient's body, the

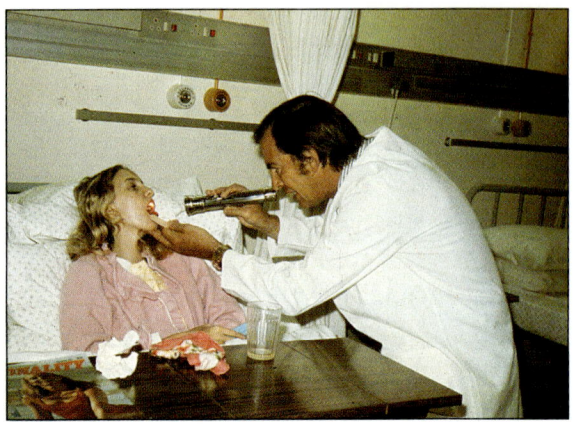

▲ **Christiaan Barnard (1922–)**, the South African surgeon who performed the first heart transplant in 1967, examining a young patient. Transplants can be given to people of any age, not just to adults.

◀ **A kidney transplant**.
Replacement organs do not always have to come from dead people. A family member is often able to give one of their kidneys to another relative because their body tissues are similar. This lowers the risk of infection. In the picture, a baby is shown after a kidney transplant. His mother, by the bed, gave one of her kidneys.

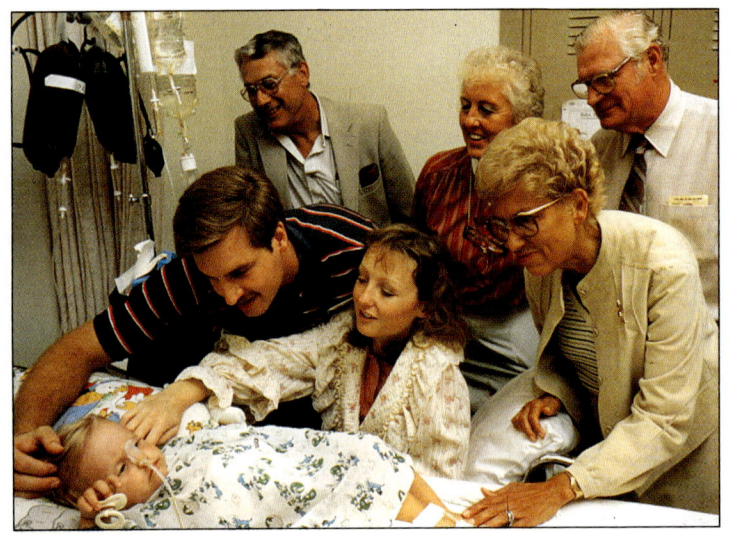

rejected kidney is taken out and another put in its place. Some people have two or three kidney transplants before they are completely well.

Replacing the heart

In 1967 a young South African surgeon called Christiaan Barnard performed the first heart transplant. His patient was a middle-aged man called Louis Washkansky, whose own heart was very damaged. The replacement heart came from a girl who had been killed in a traffic accident. At first, the operation seemed to have been successful, but eighteen days later, Washkansky died of a lung infection. The drugs he had been given to stop his body rejecting his new heart had also made it easy for him to catch infections.

Two weeks later, Barnard tried again. The patient this time was Philip Blaiberg. The operation was a success and Blaiberg survived. Since then there have been many heart transplants. The operation is still difficult and dangerous, and it is only done if no other treatment has any chance of saving the patient's life.

Questioning treatment

The pioneering work done by transplant surgeons has led to some people asking questions about transplant operations. So many advances have been made that it seems that doctors are able to do just about anything with the human body.

Could the money spent on doing

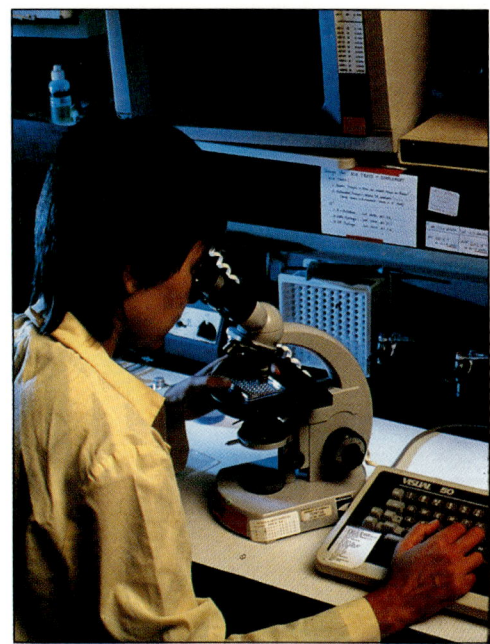

A hospital technician checks samples in a hospital laboratory in America. It is important that checks are made to make sure that the donor's tissue is compatible with that of the patient.

transplants be spent on better ways of treating illness or on more research? A heart transplant is an expensive operation and only saves one life. Would it be better to spend the money in other ways that would save many lives? Also, donor hearts for transplanting are in short supply. How do doctors decide who gets a heart transplant and who does not? Will doctors be too keen to get hearts and kidneys suitable for transplanting? Will they take hearts or kidneys from patients before they are really dead? How do doctors know that a dead person wanted their organs to be used for transplant surgery? These are difficult questions that have not yet been answered.

Time chart

Date	Pioneer	Achievement
About 400BC	Hippocrates	Starts a medical school
AD 130-200	Galen	Introduces medical ideas that last for more than 1000 years
1545	Ambroise Paré	Introduces new methods of treating wounds
1543	Andreas Vesalius	Publishes the first complete book on anatomy
1628	William Harvey	Discovers how blood circulates
1779	Humphry Davy	Discovers laughing gas, an anaesthetic
1796	Edward Jenner	Carries out the first vaccination
1842	Crawford Long	Uses ether in a surgical operation
1842	William Clark	Pulls out teeth painlessly using laughing gas
1846	William Morton	Demonstrates the use of ether in surgical operations
1847	James Simpson	Discovers chloroform, a better anaesthetic
1849	Elizabeth Blackwell	Becomes the first woman doctor
1854-6	Florence Nightingale	Nurses soldiers in the Crimean War
1860	Louis Pasteur	Invents pasteurization to kill germs
1865	Joseph Lister	Introduces antiseptics
1881	Louis Pasteur	Develops an anthrax vaccine
1882	Robert Koch	Discovers the tuberculosis bacteria
1884	Robert Koch	Discovers the cholera bacteria
1885	Louis Pasteur	Develops a rabies vaccine
1992	Sigmund Freud	Develops psychoanalysis to cure mental illness
1897	Ronald Ross	Discovers the mosquito that carries the malaria parasite

Date	Pioneer	Achievement
1909	Karl Landsteiner	Discovers blood groups
1910	Paul Ehrlich	Develops the first drug to kill bacteria
1928	Alexander Fleming	Discovers the first antibiotic, penicillin
1932	Gerhard Domagk	Develops the first sulpha drug
1940	Karl Landsteiner	Discovers the rhesus factor in blood
1940	Howard Florey and Ernst Chain	Develop a way of producing large amounts of penicillin
1954	Joseph Murray	Performs the first kidney transplant
1953	Jonas Salk	Makes a vaccine against polio
1967	Christiaan Barnard	Performs the first heart transplant

Glossary

anaesthetic: a drug used to kill pain during operations. Anaesthetics sometimes make a patient unconscious

anatomy: the science that studies how the parts of the human body are arranged and fitted together

anthrax: an infectious, fatal disease of animals such as cows and sheep caused by a germ or bacteria. It can be passed on to humans

antibiotic: a type of drug, such as penicillin, made from a mould or fungus. It is used to kill the bacteria that cause diseases

antibody: a substance produced in the blood to fight an infection. Antibodies stop the body from catching the same infection again

antiseptic: a substance that kills disease-carrying germs

artery: a large blood vessel, or tube, that carries blood from the heart to all other parts of the body

aseptic: a word meaning 'free from germs'

bacteria: very small organisms that can only be seen with a microscope. The singular is **bacterium**

bacteriology: the study of bacteria

biology: the study of living things

biologist: a scientist who studies living things

blood group: one of several types of blood into which human blood is classified

blood transfusion: giving a person new blood, after blood is lost through an accident or during an operation

chemist: a person who studies chemistry

chemistry: the science that studies what substances are made of, , how they react together, and what properties they have

chloroform: a colourless, sweet-smelling liquid that was once used as an anaesthetic, or pain killer

cholera: a disease caused by bacteria in drinking water

circulation: the movement of the blood around the body

disease: a sickness or illness

dissect: to cut up a human body or dead animal in order to study it

drug: a substance used as a medicine to cure a disease or to reduce pain

ether: a colourless, strong-smelling liquid that was once used as an anaesthetic, or pain killer

experiment: a test carried out in controlled conditions to discover something new, or to prove that an idea is correct

germ: a small organism, or bacterium, that causes a disease

malaria: a tropical disease caused by small living beings called parasites that are carried by some mosquitoes

medicine: the art of curing the sick or preventing illness

meningitis: a disease of the brain caused by a virus

mental illness: an illness in which the mind is not working properly

Nobel Prize: a prize awarded each year for important work in areas such as science, medicine, literature and international relations

parasite: an plant or animal that lives inside or on the surface of another plant or animal. It gets its food and shelter from the other plant or animal

pasteurization: a process in which liquids, especially milk, are heated to kill harmful bacteria. The word comes from the name of Louis Pasteur, the inventor of the process.

patient: a person who is being treated by a doctor

penicillin: a powerful antibiotic drug that is used to kill harmful bacteria and treat many infections

physics: the science that studies matter, the forces of nature and the different forms of energy, such as heat, light and motion

physicist: a person who studies physics

polio: abbreviation of poliomyelitis, a disease caused by a virus that weakens the muscles

psychoanalysis: a method of treating mental illness, developed by Sigmund Freud

rabies: a fatal disease of animals, especially dogs, foxes and cats, that is caused by a virus. It can be passed on to humans

rhesus factor: a substance found in the blood (85 per cent of people of European descent have rhesus factor in their blood)

science: the study of the way the world works, by using experiments and careful observation

surgery: a type of medical treatment that involves cutting the patient's body in order to repair a damaged or injured part

sulpha drug: a type of drug containing sulphur, that kills harmful bacteria

syphilis: a disease caused by bacteria and passed on through sexual contact

transplant operation: a surgical operation in which a diseased part of the body is cut out and a new part taken from another person put in its place

tuberculosis: a disease of the lungs caused by bacteria

vaccine: a substance containing antibodies that is swallowed or injected into the body to protect against disease

vaccination: the process of giving someone a vaccine either by injection or by mouth

vein: a large blood vessel that carries blood to the heart

virus: an organism smaller than a bacterium, which causes many diseases such as influenza and meningitis

Index